"This is an ambitious book and its aims – to provide a history of group analysis, to identify some of the key issues in contemporary practice and to say something about how groups might be expected to help people – are resoundingly well met. The authors expertly set out the many strands which arise in a multi-authored text of this kind and the breadth and the depth of the many well-chosen clinical examples shed light on how one might utilise that knowledge to promote insight and understanding. The contributors reflect on the original concepts and introduce some new ideas arising from their own valuable body of written work and practice illustrated with some well-chosen clinical examples. An absorbing read."

Ewa Wojciechowska, *The Institute of Group Analysis*

"This book is a declaration of love for groups and for group analysis. It tells us why groups are important, what kind of role they play in our lives and how we can use group analysis, as a specific psychotherapeutic method, to explore the inner dynamics of groups, thus helping to heal disturbed human beings. The book describes and focuses on many different aspects, thus being of great help to those, who always wanted to know, how group analysis cures and why group analysis is so efficient in doing this."

Prof. Dr. Elisabeth Rohr, *Philipps-University of Marburg, Germany and International Group Analytic Consultant (GASI)*

"This collaborative work from members of a leading group analytic network provides an invaluable exploration of how group analysis, with its understanding of the individual as a nodal point in a dynamic matrix of social, cultural, biological, and political forces, offers an effective model for a comprehensive intersectional understanding of groups and individuals in a complex, interdependent world. Covering both the underpinnings of the group analytic approach as well as contemporary developments in theory and practice, this book will engage clinicians, academics and anyone interested in the psychosocial world."

Peter Wilson, *Fitzrovia Group Analytic Practice*

W0113605

Group Analytic Therapists at Work

Group Analytic Therapists at Work is an accessible introduction to the experience of being in group analytic psychotherapy from a wide range of perspectives.

Written by members of the Group Analytic Network London, the chapters explore the history of group analysis and span key areas, including the political and the social, diversity and difference, gender and norms, and isolation and the social sphere. *Group Analytic Therapists at Work* contains discussion of themes such as group work with differing age ranges and life stages, cultural considerations, normativity, inclusion and exclusion, isolation and the internet. Each chapter provides insight from an experienced group analyst into what happens in groups, what group analysts think about while running their groups and, fundamentally, what group analysis is about.

This book will be of great interest to psychotherapists in practice and in training, group therapists and group analysts and other professionals, as well as anyone else seeking to increase their understanding of group work.

Amélie Noack is a training group analyst and a Jungian psychoanalyst. She worked in private practice, as well as teaching and supervising in the UK and abroad, was Convenor of the London Qualifying Course and Foundation Course and served on the EGATIN Committee. She now works at GRAS in Germany.

David Vincent is a group analyst and psychoanalytic psychotherapist with a Professional Doctorate from the University of Essex and worked for many years in the NHS as Consultant Adult Psychotherapist. He has been Chair of Council for the IGA and Chair of Ethics for the BPC.

Group Analytic Therapists at Work

Everyday Group Analysis

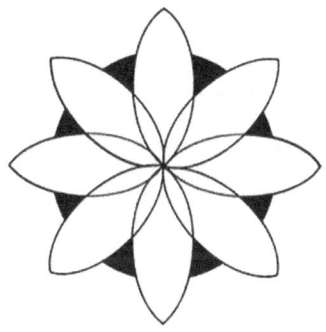

Edited by Amélie Noack and David Vincent

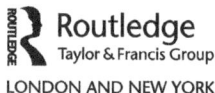 Routledge
Taylor & Francis Group

LONDON AND NEW YORK

Cover image: Cover picture by Diane Rogan. Drawing and watercolour on paper 2022. With thanks to Ballet Rambert Collaboration, The Playground. Website: www.dianerogan.com

First published 2023
by Routledge
4 Park Square, Milton Park, Abingdon, Oxon OX14 4RN

and by Routledge
605 Third Avenue, New York, NY 10158

Routledge is an imprint of the Taylor & Francis Group, an informa business

British Library Cataloguing-in-Publication Data
A catalogue record for this book is available from the British Library

ISBN: 9781032315690 (hbk)
ISBN: 9781032315683 (pbk)
ISBN: 9781003310358 (ebk)

DOI: 10.4324/9781003310358

Typeset in Times New Roman
by codeMantra

Contents

Acknowledgements

We would like to thank everybody who has been involved in the project to produce this book, everybody at Routledge, especially our editors Susannah Frearson and Saloni Singhania, and all the members at GANLondon, who contributed in various ways to it. Most of all, however, we would like to thank those people without whom this book would never have been possible, which are all the participants in all the groups, that the contributors to this book have ever worked with, may they be patients, trainees, supervisees or anybody else. We cannot name these people, but our thanks go to them all.

This book was written for everyone interested in groups, not only for interested colleagues. We hope it is written in a way that is easy and interesting to read. We wanted the book to convey our enthusiasm for groups and share the sense of excitement and joy that running groups and being in groups can bring.

Crediting sources of third-party material

We would like to thank *Group Analysis: The International Journal of Group-Analytic Psychotherapy*, for allowing the authors of this volume to quote extensively from their publication. We especially would like to thank the journal for giving permission to quote from

Azu-Okeke, O. (1993) 'Conflict in the Search for an "Individual Self" as Opposed to a Traditional "Group Self": A Consequence of Undertaking Group-Analytic Training'. *Group Analysis* 26(3): 261–268.

and from

Van der Kleij, G. (1985) 'The Group and Its Matrix'. *Group Analysis* 18(2): 102–110.

We would also like to thank Jessica Kingsley Publishers Limited for permission to reprint (permission dated 3.3.2022, ID 62225, ISN 9780857012647):

Ritchie, S. (2017) Who Helps Whom? A Group Analytic Approach to Working with Mothers and Babies in an NHS Perinatal Mental Health Service, pp. 132–143. In Celebi, M. (2017) *Weaving the Cradle: Facilitating*

Groups to Promote Attunement and Bonding between Parents, Their Babies and Toddlers. Foreword by Jane Barlow (Editor). Singing Dragon Publishers, Singing Dragon is an imprint of Jessica Kingsley Publishers: London and Philadelphia. Paperback: 248 pages; ISBN-10: 1848193114; ISBN-13: 978-1848193116

Amélie Noack and David Vincent on behalf of GANLondon

You can get in touch with GANLondon on our website www.ganlondon.net, by phone 0845 166 4154 or by sending an email to enquiries@ganlondon.net

Contributors (all contributors are member of the Institute of Group Analysis, UK)

Eugene Clerkin is a group analyst with a background in community development social work and mental health nursing. His main work has been in a crisis psychotherapy service in the NHS and his interest is in psychotherapeutic approaches that address social and financial underprivilege and extend to people hard to reach.

Sue Einhorn is a training group analyst and works in private practice. She was a Senior Lecturer in Social Work at North London Polytechnic and a therapist at the Women's Therapy Centre. Sue convened the IGA/OGRA training in St. Petersburg and currently supervises at Baobab, in Denmark, India and Singapore.

Sandra Evans is a psychiatrist, a group analyst and teacher. She worked for over thirty-five years in NHS psychiatry, mainly with older adults, has authored various papers and co-edited two books about working with older people. Since retirement, she works in private practice and in pastoral care with younger people.

Sylvia Hutchinson is a training group analyst working in private practice. Before she worked in the NHS and university settings and has been co-director of the group analytic training in Turvey. She consulted extensively to trainings in Europe and is past chairperson of the European Group Analytic Training Institutions Network (EGATIN).

Amélie Noack is a training group analyst and a Jungian psychoanalyst. She worked in private practice, as well as teaching and supervising in the UK and abroad, was Convenor of the London Qualifying Course and Foundation Course and served on the EGATIN Committee. She now works at GRAS in Germany.

Justin Phipps is a group analyst working in private practice. Before he worked as a solicitor in overseas aid and human rights. His interest is in an inter-cultural and social-anthropological approach to group analysis, and he has been involved in group analytic training and therapy in Rwanda and South Africa.

Sheila Ritchie is a training group analyst and supervisor for the IGA, working in private practice, also online both nationally and internationally. She runs a long-term group for pregnant women, mothers and babies, and is a parent-infant psychotherapist in the NHS, in a psychotherapy department and a Perinatal Parent-Infant Mental Health Service.

Diane Rogan-Sofer is a group analyst and a painter. Trained as an art therapist, she worked in a secure psychiatric setting. After working in various mental health settings, statutory NHS, HMP and voluntary sector, she now works in private practice. She still has a passion for painting and both areas of interest inform and fertilise her work.

Seda Sengun is a medical doctor trained in Turkey and a group analyst. She worked as a research assistant at the Institute of Psychiatry, then as a group analyst and supervisor in the NHS, and in private practice. Alongside her career in group analysis, she completed a doctorate in Botany.

Neil Telfer is a group analyst, originally trained in mental health nursing. He has long experience of working in the NHS, both in hospital and community settings, as well as teaching and assessing clinical practitioners. He now works in private practice. He has a passion for lyrical poetry and loves rowing.

Sarah Tucker is a training group analyst, supervisor and psychotherapist, working at Fitzrovia Group Analytic Practice. As former National Director of Training at the IGA, she developed the National Diversity Working Group: Power, Privilege and Positioning. With a deep commitment to social justice, she worked for many years with refugees and asylum seekers.

David Vincent is a group analyst and psychoanalytic psychotherapist with a Professional Doctorate from the University of Essex and worked for many years in the NHS as Consultant Adult Psychotherapist. Based on his long-standing interest in organisations, he has been Chair of Council for the IGA and Chair of Ethics for the BPC.

Introduction

What do we call what we do?

Amélie Noack and David Vincent

What do we call what we do? Do we do group analysis or group therapy? How distinguish the two? What are the differences between group psychotherapy, analytic group therapy, psychoanalytic group therapy, group psychoanalysis and group analysis?

Two recent well-received books in the UK show the difficulty: *Group Therapy – A Group-Analytic Approach* by Nick Barwick and Martin Weegman, and: *From the Couch to the Circle: Group-Analytic Psychotherapy in Practice*, by John R. Schlapobersky. An explanatory sub-title seems to be necessary.

If you could observe a session of a long-running group analytic group, you might get a rough idea of what is going on. You might get a sense that some of the group members understand what is happening, but you may also feel that the group analyst themself has not got much of an idea. This is of course the group analyst's privilege, to allow themself to become completely baffled and uncomprehending of the activities and dynamics of the group. Does it matter what the group therapist or analyst calls themself?

There is in psychotherapy a great range of distinctions about theory and technique. Often the differences are about the extent to which psychoanalysis, Jungian analysis or any other theory has influenced the particular therapy. This can be seen immediately in the real or imagined difference between, for example: group therapy, group psychotherapy and group analysis. Is one of these more psychoanalytic than the other? If so, does this matter? Or is it more important what they actually do?

Generally speaking, the principal elements distinguishing all theories of a psychoanalytic approach would be first, the importance of unconscious mental life, second, the ubiquity of the transference and countertransference, and third, arising from these two ideas, the centrality in mental life of the psychic mechanisms of splitting, denial, projection and introjection. Any group therapist working with these theories in mind could be said to be working psychoanalytically. When following a desire to make the unconscious conscious and to help the group to know itself better, a group analyst could be said to be analysing. In addition, the group analyst

DOI: 10.4324/9781003310358-1

has a continuous working interest in the social and societal factors at play in the group, how the social world gets into the individual mind, into all human relationships and into the shared life of the group.

This is not a simple matter. A member of a long-running group, an intense and rather driven man in his fifties, had what he thought was a serious heart attack. He was admitted to hospital immediately and for three days underwent numerous tests. At the end of this, the team decided that he had not had any kind of cardiac event and he was discharged. This experience led him into therapy. After some months in the group, in which he listened carefully to the others and gradually joined in, he told us, thoughtfully: "I can see that everyone else in the group has a sub-conscious. I just don't have one".

He was halfway there. This example shows how important it is for patients like this, who find self-knowledge difficult, to be treated in a group. He could see it and understand it in other group members, but not yet in himself. That was still to come.

Groups are immensely important for everybody and have great potency to change lives. Part 1 of this book will expand on this, talk about what groups are and what they are there for, why they are so important for us and why we need them. Then the specific method of group analysis will be introduced in more detail, how this method was developed and by whom, and what it has to offer. Finally, the Group Analytic Network London (GAN-London), a network of group analysts working in London, will be presented, how it came into being and how and why the professionals involved decided to work closely together and how you could join if you are interested.

Parts 2–5 will give insights into the work that group analysts do. How do group analysts work when they run their groups? How do they think about their groups? Do they think about each group member before a session? What preoccupies them afterwards when the session has finished? The various papers offer an opportunity to explore and assess how group analysts think and feel in general, when they run their groups, when they teach or when they lecture. The papers are all from past or present members of the network; some will describe work with groups in the National Health Service, while others are about work in private practice or the voluntary sector. Several papers originated as lectures, others stem from teaching and training in the UK and abroad, and a few were originally presented at GANLondon workshops. All papers have been adapted for this book, some have been written exclusively for this volume and one has been previously published.

The description of the work that group analysts do is divided up into different parts in this volume and explored under different headings. Each part starts with an introduction of the theme, explaining the topic itself in an overview and its relevance to group analysis, followed by a short synopsis of the content of each chapter.

Part 2 explores the political and social domain in group analytic work with three contributions in Chapters 4–6 respectively. Part 3 follows with the focus on the topic of 'Diversity and Difference' in Chapters 7–10. Diversity and difference are extremely important issues, currently hotly debated in the public sphere and affecting many people in their personal lives. Something similar could be said about the theme of 'Gender and norms' in Part 4, also a present-day issue with new developments regarding gender fluidity and the possibility of gender change. Part 4 presents in Chapters 11–14 differing viewpoints on how this topic can be understood in the field of group analysis. The book draws to conclusion with Part 5 and Chapters 15–18, exploring 'Isolation and the social sphere', a topic that has become even more contemporary in the past two years with the enforced isolation due to Covid-19.

The authors of these papers are all different individuals. Their histories, their way of living and working and thus their contributions here are different too. Apart from the exploration of the topic presented in each paper, these papers also offer a personal glimpse and an inkling of who these authors are as people, and how they work as professionals. Each paper is an attempt to give a truthful account of how they think and feel when working with their groups, or how they may reflect on it afterwards or in supervision, and what and how they think about group analysis in general.

More importantly, all the papers are attempts to communicate what happens in group analytic groups, where all group members, including the conductor, are working together to the same end – to offer a secure and supportive environment for learning from and with each other, to assist through social interactions the emotional development that will provide the skills needed to understand yourself and others better and to facilitate healthy relationships.

Part I

Groups and group therapy

Introduction

Most people imagine that psychotherapy, psychoanalysis or counselling usually take place in a one-to-one setting and it is not generally known that therapeutic work can also be done extremely effectively in groups. An exploration and explanation is given why groups are particularly important for human beings. Human development always happens in the context of groups, since in groups, human beings learn to relate, to communicate and to play. Groups are essential for mental health.

Group analysis, as a particular school of group psychotherapy, is described as a specific way of applying the social conception of the human being to help people understand themselves and others better and foster development and healing in the context of a therapeutic group. The history of group analysis, beginning with the founder H.S. Foulkes, is given and the development of the field over the past eighty years is outlined. A specific group of practitioners in the field, the Group Analytic Network London (GANLondon), is introduced, portraying a particular situation of working together as a group of group analysts.

Amélie Noack describes how therapy groups work and outlines the typical anxieties that occur in groups until enough trust has been developed. The benefits of learning to listen and to share with peers in a group, and the importance of the experience of mutual support in various situations of crisis in a therapy group are outlined. Finally, some important differences between group therapy and individual therapy are explained.

David Vincent, after describing a typical group therapy session along group analytic lines from an outside observer's perspective, portrays the history and development of group analysis, a specific school of thought in group therapy. Starting with the original beginnings during the Second World War and tracking the personal history of its founder S. H. Foulkes, a Jewish refugee, the interchange with developments in psychiatry and the therapeutic community movement after the war are outlined and more recent influences and developments are indicated.

DOI: 10.4324/9781003310358-2

Sue Einhorn follows with a report on a specific group of group analysts working together for more than thirty years, the GANLondon. She describes the network's development from the 1980s, including the telephone supervision network, its organisation and the way it functions on a weekly basis still today. Amélie Noack completes the chapter, outlining the experience of being a member of the network.

Chapter 1

Why groups are important and what they do

Amélie Noack

Welcome to the world of groups. This book is going to tell you why groups are important for humans, what groups are for and what groups can do. This book will also introduce you to one particular way of working with groups, called group analysis, which can be applied to working with all kinds of problems. These problems can be issues at work or of running an organisation, dealing with political matters or differences, teaching and presentation in various fields; but first and foremost, group analysis is a method used to help people with all kinds of emotional and psychological difficulties and mental health problems. In other words, groups can help to solve problems, discuss differences, support learning, but most importantly, attending a group for some time is healing – togetherness can heal.

Human beings are social beings. We do things together. We grow up in groups and we learn in groups, first in our family, then nursery and school and finally workplace. We are almost always surrounded by others, we grow and develop together.

Until the age of five, a child has to find a place in the family group. The grouping of parents and child is the basis for all group phenomena, since here the child learns how to negotiate triangular relationships. Only when there are at least three people can we speak of a group. Later, children play and learn in groups at school. Friendships are formed, but they are often not stable yet, because rivalries predominate at primary school age, and best friends can change daily. In adolescence, loyalties become more set and relationships more constant. Adolescents meet with each other in gangs or groupings that support their specific developmental needs and endorse aspects of their personality.

Groups acquire their full meaning in adulthood, because now people are able to participate in all kinds of group activity, not only at work but also in interest-groups of various kinds, for fun and leisure, cultural pursuits or creativity. As adults we are able to engage freely with our social and physical environment, maintaining, shaping and modifying it through group membership. The options are endless, from joining a book club or a political party to running events, learning to cook, looking after your grandchildren,

DOI: 10.4324/9781003310358-3

setting up a walking group or helping out in a Charity shop. These are all ways of contributing to society and participating in shaping it. Worldwide groups of any kind, like taking care of wildlife, or putting ecological or environmental concerns first, are further examples for the acknowledgement of our responsibilities as 'citizens of the world'. Adult maturity is the constructive engagement in building a better world, but it also includes recognising the effects of human destructiveness throughout the ages and addressing the suffering this has caused to other humans and the world at large.

Growing up we are exposed to countless influences from our social and physical environment, which shape who we are. As a result of these influences, we all carry around in our mind the model of a group formed by our early experiences. This model will colour our expectations of all later groups. If we have had a relatively safe early development, our expectations will be predominantly benign. If we had to grow up under difficult circumstances, neglect or abuse, or were for instance bullied at school, we will be fearful of groups later in life or even try to avoid them. But the lack of human contact – as social beings we need each other – may well result in social isolation, which, in turn, can lead to mental health problems.

The complexities of life mean that we all have to cope with the experience of disappointment and struggle and are not always able to deal with it successfully. Then it helps to talk with others. Talking in a group about those difficulties and learning to relate to one another in a safe environment, where these issues can be shared, helps to understand yourself and others better. In the process you and all other group members will grow and develop, sometimes in unexpected ways, since participation in a therapy group can also be a 'more-than-learning' experience, it can be a rediscovery of play or creativity.

Learning through being together in a group – relating

When people find themselves in any kind of group, like waiting for their child after school or queuing at a post office, they start to talk to each other, they start to relate. The person in front of you may be curious to know who you are, why you are there, what or who you are waiting for. People are curious about others, they want to relate. It might take some courage to start to speak, the other might be a complete stranger. It is daring to relate, but when you relate – you dare to be yourself. Being able to relate is so important because we only discover who we are by relating to others.

To be able to relate is important in private and public life, at work, with family and friends. We want to know how the people are, those nearest and dearest to us, how they feel, what they have experienced today. Why is your father crying; your daughter in a bad mood; or your friend angry in a way you have never seen them before? So we ask and listen – if we dare. Often it happens that the mood changes during the talking and the listening, our mood and theirs. When this happens, both parties may realise that we can grow emotionally in tandem with each other. We learn how important it is to share and to speak with each other.

We also need to communicate in public life and at work to get things done. How far is it to the next bus stop? Have you seen my spanner; the blue folder; the boss? You may discover that the person two spaces in front of you in the post office queue is saying something that moves you, even if you have never seen that person before. When we have emotional reactions to another person, some can be positive, some are emotionally uncomfortable and some may not touch us at all. In the process of relating, we discover what we feel.

Can I understand what the other is telling me, does it make sense to me? How does the other affect me? Do I like to talk to them, do I like to hear what they say? Can I listen or do I feel the need to speak all the time myself? Just by standing there in the queue, by being together with others, you hear things and you feel things, and you may learn to listen.

When we discover that others feel similar feelings to us, that they have had experiences which we can identify with, we have the experience of empathy. We feel similarly or the same. If through empathising, you discover yourself in another person, you have learnt something about yourself.

By being part of a group, we are learning from each other and with each other. This does not have to be a therapy group, quite the contrary, this happens in any group. In a group, we learn two things. We learn to be part of the group and how that feels and how we function in it, but in that group, we may also learn a skill. Playing football together you learn to follow the rules and how to get on with the other players on the field and off it, but you also are learning how to play football. During the play, the ball comes over and you kick it in a way you have never done before, you have discovered your spontaneity, you have been creative, you are playing.

Groups are a great learning environment. In groups, we learn from each other, not just from the teacher or trainer, and that is the reason why we learn best in groups. To be part of a group and to be able to use it, that is, to learn from all the various people that are part of the group is an incredible complex process. You may see how your neighbour does something – and you copy it; or you avoid it. You do not have to make all the mistakes yourself, you can learn by watching the others in the group. You notice all kinds of things, some just from the corner of your eye, some you just get the gist of. Your reactions are not always conscious, in fact, they are mostly not. A group is a very rich learning environment, there is so much going on all the time, only a small proportion of what happens is ever fully conscious. Without noticing, you are learning social skills, you are learning to speak your mind and you are learning to relate. You are growing emotionally and during this process you are becoming a fuller human being.

The need to belong – the capacity to play

Belonging is a basic human need. Healthy human beings are social beings. We like doing things in groups, because groups, and this also applies to groups at work, can be the adult equivalent to play. Work is only really emotionally satisfying if we enjoy it. When we do not enjoy the work we do, we are miserable. We may become depressed and unable to work.

The life of public figures makes this clear, especially when looking at party politics. Politicians at times seem like gangs of youngsters, where loyalties change daily, or they behave like the groupings of adolescents, behaving badly, arguing and constantly fighting for dominance with another group. But politicians also can form real work-groups and can behave like mature adults. In those work-groups, they make decisions, set goals, run the country, but also play. In the process they set taxes and make laws and organise our environment. This is hard work and they are also struggling – as we all do – to learn how to negotiate conflict in a non-violent way. As part of the wider group of world citizens, they are trying to safeguard life and are shouldering the responsibility to avoid war.

Human beings are dependent on each other. We need each other as social beings. We want to be social, we want to talk. We do invite friends for a drink or a meal. Playing an instrument alone at home is not necessarily as enjoyable as playing in an orchestra. Singing or dancing on your own or with others is a very different experience. Being part of a group can be a creative and enjoyable experience. We often watch plays in a large audience and a concert at Glastonbury is a massive group event. When things are happening at such an event within you and around you, when you are affected by others and they are by you, a 'potential space for experience' (Winnicott, 1974) opens up. In this potential space, transitional phenomena can occur or – to put it in more ordinary language – fun and play can happen. A potential space is a space for cultural experience, all those experiences which we humans can share and enjoy sharing with each other, because the sharing itself becomes a creative experience.

Group therapy – togetherness can heal

The Institute of Group Analysis (IGA) was set up in the 1970s to train people interested in learning how to conduct the kind of groups that would promote the psychological development of the people in these groups. One of the founder members was S. H. Foulkes, a German Jewish psychiatrist and psychoanalyst, who had arrived in Britain in 1933 from Nazi Germany. He was one of the first clinicians to develop a method for group psychotherapy and described his method as a treatment of the group, by the group, including the conductor. In contrast to other methods of therapy, in group analysis, the conductor or the therapist is also, like every other group member, subject to the emotional impact of the group process and the necessity for change. Foulkes called his method group analysis in contrast to individual analysis. The IGA teaches, studies and cultivates his tradition.

Starting therapy

Usually, you have had a few sessions with the group therapist who explains it all. Then you find yourself in the group for the first time. Anxiety is high and you are not the only one wondering if the group is safe. Can you trust this group? How much can you say? How do you engage with the others? Anxieties and fear of rejection predominate. Everybody wonders: How to relate to each other? What is allowed in the group? What belongs here and what not? At the beginning, these questions are often directed at the group conductor, who – if they do their work well – will redirect them to the group: What does the group think? Everybody is asked to be part of the group and to contribute. This is daunting. Do you dare to speak your mind? Feelings of insecurity and lack of confidence are often triggered. The question is, can these feelings be tolerated and expressed by people in the group or do they need to be denied?

When people begin to feel safe and can share what they feel, they gain confidence and start to address other, more worrying issues. When people feel safe enough, they loosen up, relax and may get 'worse'. That means they may dare to take more time or interrupt someone speaking. Acting out in other ways, like missing a session, may occur when some anger could not be verbalised. All in all, people are using the group well to explore and share difficult issues from the past or the present that need to be talked about. Now people have learnt that they are not the only ones who suffered loss or had painful and hurtful experiences.

At first these feelings may seem unbearable and people come into contact with shame, anger and guilt, but group members are often profoundly moved when they hear about the difficulties of others. Anxieties concerning madness and badness, sexuality, illness and destructiveness may come up at this stage. When something scary comes up there is a need to talk about it. The fact that a difficult issue can be verbalised is usually a sign that now it 'can' be talked about.

There may be a fear to get lost in all this 'primitive stuff' and this evokes a desire to disengage or to run away. The group may seem to be worse, but all the difficult stuff is in actual fact an indication that the people in the group are allowing themselves to be dependent and to regress. In short, the group is functioning well therapeutically and is doing valuable work. Before and after breaks, the group may feel let down and angry that there were or will be no more sessions for some time. Breaks cause anxiety, but each break is also a challenge to grow up a bit more and to claim again some independence. In addition, each break is an opportunity for development. After a break, people may have changed or new developments may be visible and other group members may comment on it.

If a group has become a safe environment and works well, the individuals in the group are able to develop in their own pace and in accordance with their own potential and their own needs. When a group member feels ready to leave, the whole group discusses their readiness. Sometimes they change their mind and stay on for longer, sometimes not. It is tremendously important that the leaver is sure to have the backup of the whole group when they depart to begin a new chapter and the next stage in their life.

Supporting each other through crisis

It is frightening to be a newcomer to a group. The experience of anxiety due to insecurity and not feeling safe goes hand in hand with the expectation of rejection or even attacks from others in the group. We all know the feelings connected with this experience. It happens when we first start school or walk into a party, where we do not know anybody, or when we join any group which is new to us.

Before developing a sense of belonging to a group, every newcomer has to face this state of 'paranoid' anxiety, an emotional experience full of fears and expectations. Joining a group is a frightening experience. In order to negotiate this frightening situation, every newcomer to a therapy group needs a firm connection with the group conductor. The conductor is your ally and – in your fantasy at least – you can hold on to their hand or hide behind them. It is important to acknowledge this bond or alliance to enable the newcomer to overcome their fear of joining the group, and usually this has been discussed in detail in the preliminary meetings. It will make the prospective newcomer feel safe enough to tolerate the experience. In addition, other group members may reach out to the newcomer by sharing how they felt when they originally joined the group. The newcomer can also ask how this was for the older group members, if they have the courage to do so.

At some point in time, the newcomer will need to tell the other group members why they decided to join the group, what they are expecting to gain from being part of it. Usually, we decide to start therapy, when we realise that something is not quite right in our life and that we want this to change. There will be change eventually, change that might surprise even yourself.

Therapy really is a means to get the necessary help and support to make change happen. But in order to get the support, you need to start to talk. You need to tell people what bothers or worries you, or in a more poetic language, what it is that 'ails you', what makes you ill or ill at ease. You will need to talk and share your story, you will need to open up and communicate. This, in turn, will enable the other group members to listen and hear who you are and eventually understand you. Group members are usually curious to get to know a new group siblings. They may ask for your story or support you in verbalising it in other ways.

One of the reasons why so many people fear or hesitate to join a therapy group, may be that they had fearful experiences in their early family life. We all carry around in our minds the very complex model of a group formed by our early experiences in our first family group. This internal model is activated when we join a group and will colour our expectations, as well as trigger so-called transferences. Transferences are experiences where another member of the group appears to treat you like your mother or father or another member of your family. You may feel put down as you did by your mother or feel angry in the same way as your father made you feel. Since the other group members are actually strangers and do not belong to your family, such situations are excellent opportunities to talk this though or 'work this through', as we say in analytical language. Transferences that appear in the group are based on earlier experiences in life and part of the work of group analysis is to recognise them and work them through. This, in turn, helps to understand what happened in the past and supports you to overcome the old experience. Other group members will have had similar experiences, they already may know some of their transference reactions to others in the group and they can help you with recognising and understanding this complicated situation.

Learning to talk and to listen

Everything that goes on in the group is important. Tell the group if you observe something going on, which nobody else seems to notice. Talk to the group about how you feel, say if someone makes you feel welcome and understood or when another seems not to listen or you feel they are behaving in a rejecting way. Everything is significant, it has some meaning and needs to be communicated. Problems often arise because we did or do not dare to talk about it. Dare to speak your mind, even if another group member reacts with anger or discomfort. All of this can be talked about.

As a member of the group you learn to relate, you learn to listen and you learn to witness. People's life stories are often difficult and in a therapy group, painful things can be talked about, maybe for the first time. When someone reveals an upsetting experience, they want to be listened to, but they may also afterwards want to hear how you felt in response. They want to know that now they are not alone with their suffering any longer, but that there are others who share the load. Things that you may hear from your group members can be upsetting and distressing, some will be even hair-raising. By witnessing what happened and by empathising with the experience you lift some of the heavy weight of their shoulders. Not all lives are smooth journeys, most lives are a mixture of pleasure and pain, and in the group, you will also hear some heart-warming stories. There will be laughter too, pleasure and fun. People cry and laugh in therapy groups!

We all have bad days and get moody at times. Perhaps we have not slept well or did miss the bus. Our partner forgot to get milk or has told us – again – we needed to lose weight. Something upset us, we are annoyed and arrive in the group in a grumpy mood. Then one of your group siblings says the 'wrong' thing and you snort derisively. Others may point out that you behaved dismissively, you feel got at and respond aggressively: 'This group isn't working. I think I should leave'.

Obviously, this needs to be talked through, and if the group is too stunned to start this, the group conductor will initiate the process. Group members usually feel incredibly loyal to the group and to other group members and do not like it when an individual or, like here, the group-as-a-whole is attacked. The result of the shock is at first often a stunned silence, but then generally moves on into flight-fight mode. This means some group members pull back defensively, while others will attack, in turn, which can feel rather scary. How the group manages to resolve the conflict depends very much on the maturity of the group and in the last resort the group conductor is available to lend a helping hand to enable everybody to understand how disagreements like this arise and how they can be settled.

Preparing to leave

One of the major struggles for group members is leaving the group. Leaving is an extremely crucial happening for human beings since it brings all earlier leavings and separations and their idiosyncrasies to the fore. Separation is an enormous stumbling block in psychological development for every human being, beginning with birth, when we leave the comforting all-around environment of the womb, over starting nursery or school and countless more separations in between, to eventually dying and leaving this world again.

Each separation moves us on and forward in our psychological development, if we can bear the loss and allow ourselves to grieve what we leave behind. Leaving is only ever successful, when we can acknowledge and accept that we gained from what we leave behind. We can only separate from a positive object or experience, the negative cannot be left behind, since it cannot be mourned. To arrive at the point of readiness for separation often takes more time than originally expected. Individuals in the group will arrive in their own time at the point when they are ready to leave the group. Then it is essential that the decision can be talked about in depth with the whole group. Timing and reasons, as well as future plans and endeavours need to be aired and tested for reliability. As emphasised before, it is tremendously important that the leaver has the full backup of the group, when they leave to start a new chapter in their life.

How to decide: group or individual therapy

We live in a complex world and coping with the complexities is not always easy. After an accident or the loss of a loved one, people may find themselves in difficulties or unable to cope and may develop mental health problem. Many people know these days that therapy or counselling are available to help them deal with such a situation or to support them through crisis after an emergency and may have even been referred for individual counselling. Much fewer people know that group therapy is also available and an equally valid form of therapy.

Greater visibility

Group therapy can address similar issues as individual therapy, like relationship problems, depression or anxiety, but the group situation is a much more suitable therapeutic medium for difficulties relating to social anxieties, which are on the rise nowadays. In a group, there are many more people present who can listen, hear and support you, and the scenario is wider and richer than in the individual setting. Projection and transferences are also distributed amongst many and appear not only in relation to the therapist. The group conductor may well be seen as a parental figure or as the super-ego, and this arouses particular expectations, fears and wishes, but they vary for everybody in the group. The working through of these projections and transferences by others in the group can be observed in the group setting, and this visibility helps people to understand their internal objects and current relationships better. Problems of authenticity and authority can also clearly be seen in a group. If you cannot be authentic and take possession of your own personal authority in a group, the other group members will sense this and challenge you.

Challenging authority

With the support of others in the group, a remark or a statement by the therapist can be questioned and relativised, something that can never happen in individual therapy. For instance, group members may support one of their group siblings by challenging the therapist's view. Such an event has enormous potential. It may change a lifelong need for the security of parental figures and the resulting submission to their authority. It is striking how much easier group members take challenges or criticism from their fellow members rather than from the group conductor. Peer insights can be questioned much more easily, but also accepted with less difficulties – we basically learn best from our peers. New ways of behaviour can then be tried out amongst equals.

Valuing the social and diversity

As said before, problems originating in the family of origin are not necessarily given enough consideration in individual therapy due to the focus on internal psychic dynamics. In group therapy, public, social and political aspects and their influences are always considered in addition to the personal.

With its variety of personal backgrounds, including class, sexual orientation, ethnicity or culture, the group setting provides a rich tapestry of experience akin to that found in the wider social environment today. The possibility to encounter and negotiate diversity is essential for the societies we live in, where multi-cultural groupings are more and more prevalent. The multi-cultural groupings in our societies come with a high potential for insecurity, because society as a whole now shares a smaller common ground due to the underlying differences and cultural variations. This generates a greater general base of anxiety and aggression.

The differences need to be recognised, addressed and thought about in the therapy group, so that the deep and often unconscious mutual cultural deprecations can be recognised and acknowledged. The necessary process of recognition and acceptance in a group fosters mutual understanding and acceptance and promotes a value system that embraces diversity and invites otherness.

Groups are the natural environment for human beings. They are necessary for our development. Groups are frightening, but this fear can be addressed in the group since projections and transferences are visible and shared out. In groups, the therapist can be questioned and challenged since groups emphasise sibling relationships. Groups provide diversity and differences and can make you more mature, since they promote an awareness of human destructiveness and suffering. Groups force you to be authentic and develop authority and groups have enormous potential, which has not only therapeutic significance but also social, political and environmental relevance.

Chapter 2

History and development of group analysis

David Vincent

Every day, wherever you are, at any time of the day, there will almost certainly be group therapy going on somewhere near you. A small group of people, perhaps seven or eight, will be sitting in a circle of chairs in a quiet room, talking. In one way, they will be doing together what people have, of course, always done: trying to understand what is going on around them, and within them, by speaking to others and asking to be heard, for advice, for friendship and for understanding from one another. In another way, they will be doing group therapy, which concerns us here, and a different, very particular type of conversation will be taking place. The people in the therapy group are probably troubled in some way, grieving, depressed or anxious. They are looking for help with this, and they have ended up together, here, near where you are standing or sitting right now, talking to one another about what ails them. If this is group therapy, then there will, almost certainly, be a group leader with them: a psychotherapist, psychiatrist or counsellor. If you could now, unseen, observe them, what would you see?

You might first of all notice that there is an overall feeling in the group. Perhaps it is quiet and thoughtful, or angry, tense and uneasy. You would see that most of the time the members of the group seem to listen to one another but that there will also be times in the group when people shout and laugh and interrupt one another. You would see that they seem, for the most part, to take it in turns to speak, but that some are almost always silent. You would then see, after observing them for a while, that the mood and atmosphere continually change, that some people are always much quieter than others, that some get angry very easily, and that others are overcome at times with anxiety or sadness. You would notice that the group leader appears to be calm and thoughtful and speaks only rarely. You might have a vague feeling that this is not easy for the leader, and that they are often, beneath the surface, struggling to stay attentive or to listen and be patient. When they speak it is almost always to comment on, or talk to, the group as a whole, and only more rarely do they speak to, or about, individual members of the group.

DOI: 10.4324/9781003310358-4

If you watched them to the end you might be surprised to see the group leader stop the group quite suddenly, at the end of the allotted time, which you might notice is nearly always ninety minutes. Some of the group members would jump up, and leave immediately, others would take their time, and might linger at the door of the building to talk. If you were there a week later, you might see the exact same process take place again: the group leader would be quiet, the angry people would be angry again and the lingerers would wait at the door for their fellow group members at the end of the session. If by any chance you could observe this group for a long time, you would be surprised to see, all being well, that, in spite of everything seeming to be the same from week to week, a very slow, almost imperceptible, change for the better would be taking place, in the feeling of the group as a whole, and in some, or perhaps all, of the individuals. It might be surprising because it would be almost impossible, no matter how carefully you observed them, to see how, or why, that change took place. Nevertheless, change it did. So, every day, around you, something like this is going on. It is group therapy.

There are many different kinds of group therapy in the world. Some are the same, some very similar to others, but with radically different language, and there are others that are apparently quite different. Most of them are, however, roughly similar in practice, if not in theory. In other words, in and between different group psychotherapy approaches, as in all the social and medical sciences, there may be widely different theoretical and technical explanations for what, to the innocent observer, may look like the same phenomena. Within the range of possible approaches, the kind of group therapy that this book is concerned with is known as group analysis. This is group therapy as it is taught at the Institute of Group Analysis, where all of the contributors to this book were trained, and where many of them work, teach and supervise.

Group analysis – the beginning

Group analysis began to take form in the Second World War. Although there had been some attempts before the war to develop group methods of treatment in psychiatry, mostly in the United States, and a little in the United Kingdom, it was systematically developed during the war and then used to treat soldiers returning from battle, who were suffering from 'shell-shock' or 'battle-fatigue' or what is now known as Post-Traumatic Shock Disorder (PTSD), by army psychiatrists, in particular by those working in a military hospital in Birmingham called Northfield. The military situation at this point in the Second World War was dire, and there was a great need to return any suitable soldiers to active duty and to treat the remaining casualties as quickly as possible. The first version of this hospital treatment service at Northfield was set up by Wilfred Bion and John Rickman. It ran for six weeks and was then closed down, following institutional problems, to be replaced by another scheme run largely by S.H. Foulkes and his colleagues (Harrison, 2000). In this second version, there was a great deal of innovation and experiment over the next few years, right up until the end of the war. In particular, Foulkes and his colleagues developed small group psychotherapy, in the form of what later became known as group analysis, as a method of treatment, first of all, for soldiers with PTSD (Foulkes, 1948).

At Northfield, there were at the same time also the beginnings of the clinical practice in a number of methods, like art and music therapy, the 'large group' and community meetings, intensive psychiatric nursing and milieu therapy. Many of the staff went on to work in various ways after the war in further developments in psychiatry (Bion, 1961; Pines, 1985).

At the end of the war, there was tremendous social ferment: the 'servicemen's election', the first Labour Government, the mass movement and resettlement of refugees and the rehabilitation of returning prisoners of war, the 1944 Education Act and the hard-fought establishment of the National Health Service. All of these affected the gradual development of group psychotherapy and group analysis. But particularly in the treatment of neurosis and personality disorder within National Health Service psychiatry, there was an obvious easy transition of group and social treatment methods from military to civilian settings through both treatment techniques and personnel.

Group analysis – the background

There were of course many other influences on the growth and establishment of group analysis before, during and after the Second World War. Foulkes himself embodied and brought to group analysis a wide range of important ideas. He was German: a neurologist, psychiatrist and psychoanalyst. In his medical training, he was very influenced by Goldstein, the neurologist who developed the concept of 'holistic' neurology, seeing the part in relation to the whole, the neurological symptom in relation to the patient as a person. This combined with another influence from the 'Gestalt' psychologists, who analysed perception with a view to understanding all sight as an act of relating the foreground to the background. In time, this gave rise to the important basic understanding in group analysis, that the 'figure' always stands in relation to the 'ground' as the 'individual' stands in relation to the 'group'.

Foulkes had joined the German Army in 1917 at the age of eighteen and served in a signals regiment. After the war, he took his medical and psychiatric training and then in 1928, he went to Vienna to train as a psychoanalyst. His training analyst was Helene Deutsch. In 1930, after qualification, he returned to Frankfurt to become head of the new clinic for psychoanalysis. Foulkes and his colleagues began to work with sociologists from the Frankfurt School for Social Research, and this became another important influence on the subsequent development of Group Analysis. These sociologists, like Theodor Adorno, Herbert Marcuse, Karl Mannheim and Erich Fromm, began to look to psychoanalysis for help in understanding the move of the German working class away from socialism and trade unionism and into the Nazi Party. Traditional Marxist and socialist theory suggested that this was against their own interests as workers. Perhaps psychoanalysis could help to explain this. This led a number of them into personal psychoanalysis and a life-long interest in combining social and psychological theory.

Many of the sociologists went as refugees to the United States and some of them reformed the Frankfurt School of Social Research into the New School of Social Research in New York. Most notable of the refugees from Frankfurt were perhaps Theodor Adorno with his famous study 'The Authoritarian Personality', and Herbert Marcuse with a series of works that were very influential in the 1960s, like 'One Dimensional Man' and 'Eros and Civilisation', attempted to combine revolutionary socialism and psychoanalysis (Adorno & Frankel-Brunswick, 2019; Marcuse, 2002). The best known in this group was Erich Fromm, who wrote about both in a series of works in the United States (Fromm, 1970, 1999). His wife, Frieda Fromm-Reichman, was also a psychoanalyst, who joined Erich in the United States and worked for many years at Chestnut Lodge, the famous psychoanalytic hospital, where also Harold Searles worked (Hornstein, 2000; Searles, 1986b). Others from Frankfurt came as refugees to Britain. The sociologists Karl Mannheim and Norbert Elias worked in London and Leicester, and Elias in particular continued his working friendship with Foulkes in Britain (Elias, 1994).

Foulkes – his personal history

Foulkes was Jewish and in 1933 he and his young family left Germany to escape Nazi persecution. On the invitation of Ernest Jones, who was then the president of the British Psychoanalytic Society, he came to London, where he joined the group led by Anna Freud at the British Psychoanalytic Society and took a British medical qualification. In 1939, as potential patients left London for fear of the bombing, Foulkes moved to Exeter to work as a psychotherapist in a private psychiatric practice. While there, he made his first attempt at group therapy, bringing his individual patients together in the waiting room of the practice. Something important had just started.

In 1942, Foulkes joined the British Army Medical Corps as a psychiatrist and was posted to Northfield Hospital where he worked for the duration of the war. To chart his development over this period, it is interesting to compare two of his early papers. In 1937, he wrote 'On Introjection' as his membership paper for the British Psychoanalytical Society (Foulkes, 1990, pp. 57–82). It is a thorough and well-referenced contribution to classic psychoanalytic literature and for the most part very conventional. However, at one point in the paper he quotes, approvingly, the psychoanalyst Paul Schilder, whom he had known in Vienna:

The new-born child has a world, and probably even the embryo has. The borderline will not be rigorously defined, and one may see part of the body in the world and part of the world in the body. In other words, from the point of view of adult thinking the body will be projected into the world, and the world will be introjected into the body.

(Foulkes, 1990, p. 76)

The word 'group' could of course be substituted for 'world' in this quotation. Schilder in fact went as a refugee to the United States later and while there began himself to develop small group therapy. At this point though, in 1937, Foulkes was obviously very taken by this complex thought and it perhaps unconsciously informed his changing thinking.

The work at Northfield helped Foulkes and his colleagues to develop small group therapy and group analysis, and he refers to this time frequently in his writing, notably in his first book (Foulkes, 1948). But already in 1946 he had presented a second paper to the British Psychoanalytical Society, this time about his work at the hospital. This is a very different sort of paper from his first, busy and enthusiastic, very concerned with the development of his own ideas and emphasising the need to be careful about

introducing a preconceived theory into the observation of facts.

(Foulkes, 1990, p. 129).

Instead, he insisted:

We must be in spontaneous contact with a life situation.

(ibid.)

This eventually became a necessarily not very well described or theorised tenet of group analysis. You might say that every group takes place primarily – or even only – in the present moment, when it is at its most alive.

The development of group analysis

Foulkes by now had around him several colleagues, more or less a group, who gradually took on the work of developing and advancing group analysis (Pines, 1982). Together they formed the Group Analytic Practice (GAP), the Group Analytic Society (GAS), and later the Institute of Group Analysis (IGA), who began the training courses. There was a great deal of interaction, as well as rivalry between group analysis and other movements in the field.

Under the influence of Robin Skynner, an early group analyst, the Institute of Family Therapy formed (Skynner, 1976). At the Tavistock Clinic, by 1948, part of the new National Health Service, group methods flourished, influenced by the work of Wilfred Bion and later by Henry Ezriel. The Tavistock Institute of Human Relation had separated organisationally from the Tavistock Clinic at the start of the NHS (Bion, 1961; Ezriel, 1980; Trist & Murray, 1990).

The therapeutic community movement, influenced by the Northfield Experiment, began to have a great impact through Maxwell Jones, who had run a rehabilitation hospital at Dartford during the war and then the Henderson Hospital. Tom Main was also a leading figure. He had been at Northfield Hospital and later became the director of the Cassell Hospital in Richmond (Barnes, 1968; Manning, 1989). The Henderson specialised in working with sociopathic disorders and the Cassell was a 'psychoanalytic hospital'. Both these organisations were very important for the NHS through their publications and through the many members of staff they trained, and who later went on to work elsewhere (Barnes, 1968).

Over the years, group analysis was influenced by all of these developments and by many others. The consequent developments, arguments and disagreements were described later by Earl Hopper, Farhad Dalal, Morris Nitsun and John Schlapobersky (Dalal, 1998, 2002; Hopper, 2003a, 2003b, 2012; Nitsun, 1996; Schlapobersky, 2016). These follow on from Foulkes' own writing about the group analytic tradition (Foulkes, 1948, 1964; Foulkes & Anthony, 1957).

This account of group analysis and its development is a necessarily simplified account of what is in fact a rich and complex movement in social and psychological thought. Group analysis is only one strand in this, but it is an important one, since it has many long-term consequences for the health of individuals, groups and societies. Group analysts, like other psychotherapists, work in both public and private settings, teaching and training. Some of them establish themselves in both formal and informal practices in order to share and trade referrals and other group-analytic work, as generally speaking it is helpful to have a good mixture of patients in treatment groups. Group analysis tends to be an urban pursuit.

Chapter 3

The Group Analytic Network London

Sue Einhorn and Amélie Noack

Setting up the network

In 1984, the only private clinical practice for group analysts existed at Montague Mansions, just off Baker Street. All the trainees of the Institute of Group Analysis (IGA), which had been formed in 1971, attended their therapy groups with the founding members of the IGA at this practice.

Qualifying as a group analyst and setting up in private clinical practice, which included running analytic groups, was somewhat daunting. In 1984, two of the early trainees to qualify at the IGA, Michael Kelly and Anne Mhlongo (later Morgan), decided to set up a local network for support and referrals. They had both worked in therapeutic communities and very much valued the ethos of the collective approach. They wanted the Group Analytic Network London (GANLondon) to be a growing network of colleagues, who would meet together for support and referrals. In contrast to the Group Analytic Practice in Montague Mansions, they would not take responsibility for a property or share a physical clinic space, but every member of the network would have to take care of their own consulting room, somewhat like a cottage industry. Soon after Gill Barratt joined them, and in 1987 Sheila Ernst did too. The network grew further when Farhad Dalal became a member in 1991 and Sue Einhorn in 1992.

The early meetings were sporadic and happened approximately once every six weeks. By 1992, however, we were meeting weekly and now could think about referrals and include clinical discussions of our work, together with the more practical administration of the network. Our commitment was to not exceed our membership beyond the number of groups we could support. By this time, we were supporting six mixed groups, two women's groups, and one couple's group. When Anne Morgan left in 1996 to emigrate to South Africa, Sandra Evans and Michael Lodrick joined. Ten years later Sylvia Hutchinson became a member, Norman Vella in 2008, David Vincent in 2010 and Amélie Noack in 2011.

All members of GANLondon were active members of the IGA in London, working on committees or chairing them and teaching or supervising

DOI: 10.4324/9781003310358-5

trainees on the Qualifying Course. Sheila and Anne also had strong links with the Manchester Block Training in group analysis that emerged in the late 1980s. Michael Kelly was very active as a trainer in Ireland, especially Belfast. All of us were deeply involved with the development of group analysis and also continued the group analytic tradition of learning about other cultures through EGATIN (European Group Analytic Training Institutes Network), where Sylvia and Amélie were very active, and EATGA (European Association of Transcultural Group Analysis), where Sue was engaged. Most of us were also members of GASI, The Group Analytic Society (international), and enthusiastic attendees at their international Symposium every third year.

One of the endeavours of GANLondon was to move the location of private therapy away from Northwest London, further into the East. In the early years, network members practised primarily in Haringey and Hackney and consciously focused on developing connections with referral sources in their areas and further into East London. To support this development, we initiated a termly event, entitled 'The Psyche-Soma', and invited local colleagues from different professions to join us to discuss the issues raised. We invited doctors, chiropractors, homeopaths, counsellors from GP practices, social workers, psychiatrists and psychologists along with others. Each approach would demonstrate how it understood and managed the Psyche-Soma and discuss similarities and differences. We learnt a great deal from each other and also gradually enriched our presence as GANLondon locally.

The early years of GANLondon were founded on the therapeutic community ethos, where there was a link between one's personal life and one's work life. Our weekly meetings required the confidentiality and trust of a clinical space, but over the years this led to a more personal connection, which also included our partners and family. Each year we would spend a weekend away together, free from work. We would be walking and cooking together with our partners, including some children – a sort of therapeutic retreat. As GANLondon expanded over the years, this evolved into an annual social event, which excluded partners but included colleagues, also from other areas of work. We were moving away from the cottage industry model into a more professional network. The Psyche-Soma meetings were long gone and by 1998, we were organising annual workshops to show others how we worked. Many of the themes and papers in this book have arisen from these workshops. True to our roots these early workshops took place in Hackney, at the Homerton Hospital, at East London College and other local venues. The annual GANLondon workshop still takes place today, but it now takes place at the IGA in Swiss Cottage as our membership has grown and changed.

The telephone supervision network

In 1994, Anne and Sheila, who had been working on the Manchester Block training together, decided to start another venture and set up the

GANLondon Telephone Supervision Network. This was initially for graduates from the Manchester Training Course, who had been used to telephone supervision between their training blocks. Once qualified, their need for supervision continued, but these colleagues lived far from each other and so the idea of the Telephone Supervision Network was born. One supervisor would meet in a telephone conference with four supervisees on a fortnightly basis. The hours of supervision were designed to meet the requirements of the UKCP (United Kingdom Council for Psychotherapy). When a third supervision group was needed the following year, Sue joined the Telephone Supervision Network. In addition to the fortnightly telephone supervision, there were three days each year when the entire Telephone Supervision Network would meet together face to face in London. On this day, a shared lunch was provided and in addition to the small supervision groups, everybody would also come together for a group discussion, where one of the supervision groups would present a previously prepared topic.

The Telephone Supervision Network continues today, but now using acceptable video platforms instead of the telephone. The supervisory work supports and enriches colleagues throughout the country. Members working in similar settings, but in different areas of the UK, are able to explore different ways of meeting the challenges of, for instance, groups in PD departments, psychology departments, closed wards, prisons and private practice. More experienced members offer support to new members, helping them to find jobs or begin to work in private practice. Over the years, the depth of the supervision is enriched, as new members join and others leave, in this particular application of the slow-open model of group analysis itself.

The associates membership scheme

By the early 2000s, Anne had long gone and Michael and Gill were considering retirement. We were thinking about the future of GANLondon, and Sue Einhorn suggested to initiate an Associates Scheme.

Several colleagues had said how isolated they felt after qualification, since unless IGA members are working in clinics or voluntary settings, they have few links with other group analysts once they graduate. Being part of GANLondon would offer a way to remain connected to a network of colleagues, especially for those who were working as clinicians both privately and in the public sector and would not want to become full members. Others did not intend to set up in private practice, but still wanted a group analytic environment to discuss their clinical or organisational work. It felt very important to maintain links with colleagues working in such different settings.

An associate can attend our yearly workshops and two of our weekly meetings per term. In addition, they are invited to our annual social event, which they may use to extend their own professional networks. Being an associate allows group analysts to get to know us better, especially if they wish to eventually become a full member. This option gives everybody a chance to meet before the profound commitment of the weekly meetings. It also allows us to consider our capacity, since we continue to be concerned about the number of private groups we can support.

Another purpose of the associates project was to offer a link for those members who were preparing to retire or, indeed, had retired. It offered the option to remain connected to GANLondon, attend twice per term if they so wished, continue to attend our workshops and meet up with us again at the annual social.

These different relationships in the network may seem complicated, but the associates scheme has enriched GANLondon by keeping us linked to members working in the health service and, in return, offers them a network they can belong to.

GANLondon today

After discussing any new referrals, the main part of the weekly meeting is devoted to one of us presenting our clinical work for discussion. The person presenting may be a full member but may also be an associate member presenting an issue from their own clinical practice. It is important to state that we all work together in that we supervise our clinical work collectively.

At the moment, we are eight full GANLondon members. We support each other to conduct thirteen private groups. Once each term, a meeting is scheduled for administrative responsibilities, which includes invitations for the social and the workshop, but also the planning of the annual workshop. We continue to meet each week and we have a chairperson who facilitates each meeting. This function rotates, since GANLondon is not formally hierarchically structured, so a therapeutic community ethos continues to a certain degree. Each year we organise an annual away day, where future planning for GANLondon is on the agenda, but this day also offers a space for more difficult personal issues between ourselves to be aired and discussed.

The history of GANLondon can also be seen as an example to set up a private clinical practice in a group analytic way. We do support our members setting up new private groups, but over the years, we have also been able to pass on groups to the next generation, when a colleague retires or dies – sometimes unexpectedly. It is in fact a shock when this happens – to people in the respective group and to us as colleagues – and sadly we have experienced this several times. We therefore also carry responsibility within the Network for each other's professional wills.

Becoming and being a GANLondon member

As stated before, many trainees during the 1990s attended their therapy group at Montague Mansions at the Group Analytic Practice (GAP). For aspiring group analysts, this was the place to be, since all prominent group analysts were working there. A busy practice, with lots of comings and goings, many trainees dreamed of working there one day too. After qualification, however, the idealising transferences often had crumbled and working as part of GAP was not necessarily what was wanted.

In the past, trainees would have met GANLondon members during training, either as teachers or supervisors. If you wanted regular contact with colleagues and the option to discuss your work together, GANLondon was the port of call and it is still possible to become a member today. After an initial – friendly but nevertheless daunting – interview, it is possible to become an associate member and you can remain an associate member for several years, if meeting every week is not an option.

Being a full member includes the regular commitment of meeting once every week for ninety minutes. Ninety minutes are the group analytic hour, and this timeframe applies to all sessions at the IGA, to therapy, median or large groups, as well as seminars and committee meetings, and it also applies to the weekly meeting of GANLondon. After discussing referrals, members present their group on a rotational basis. With admin meetings and associates timetabled in, each full member presents at least every second term. Usually one or two associate members can join the weekly work presentations to listen and learn, but there are some meetings when only full members can attend. This is the case when training group analysts present their twice-weekly group. They have to safeguard the boundaries in order to protect the confidentiality of training candidates in their group. But there are also training group analysts in GANLondon who decide to take their work for supervision outside of GANLondon.

Members present their own group(s) in these meetings, but since they also hear the presentations of everybody else, full members have a good sense how their colleagues work in their therapy groups. When a GANLondon member, say, gets ill unexpectedly, it is perfectly possible to ask a colleague for support. GANLondon members hold the professional will for other members and can contact individual patients if necessary or even organise a replacement for a group conductor who is seriously ill. While this may create some friction when the rightful conductor returns, for instance, the group complaining that they were happier with the replacement's way of running the group, this again has to be understood analytically. The complaint is a creative way to express the group's anger towards their conductor for leaving them with a complete stranger.

At GANLondon, every member pays membership fees, with associates paying a third of the full fee. These moneys pay for the administrator, who attends admin meetings and covers the organisation for the workshops. It also finances the yearly social gathering and pays for the away day.

Through meeting regularly and sharing their work, GANLondon members also experience each other's way of working. This makes it easier to refer patients, who may need specific skills or a particular approach. To be able to say 'I know this colleague and their way of working' or 'You would fit well into that group' makes patients feel held and well taken care of.

Working so closely with each other, a degree of sensitivity for the idiosyncrasies of other colleagues develops. At the meetings, people encounter each other primarily on a 'persona' level, a protective and sometimes defensive stratum of the personality, which may cover insecurities and inferiorities, which individuals may prefer to keep private. Not everybody favours close relationships or feels comfortable with disclosing vulnerabilities in a work group. Being a member of GANLondon, however, means that over the years, people get to know each other personally very well and indeed develop friendships.

Being part of a network of colleagues is helpful in many ways. The support of others, who know you and your specific skills, is supportive in a fundamental way. In addition to the usual formal supervision that most group analysts attend, being part of a network gives a sense of belonging and place, as well as being part of a greater unit. It allows to draw on the resources of experienced colleagues and to make use of the variety of experience offered in the network. To be in touch with the diversity of ways of working and appreciate the enrichment based on the input of others is mutually rewarding. To share the difficulties and the joy of working with groups with each other employs one of the basic principles of group analysis. The experience of togetherness is extremely advantageous for practising group analysts, it is a reminder of what groups are for. The benefits of this kind of personal and professional contact and support are invaluable.

Part 2

The political and the social

Introduction

The political and the social domains are both basic constituents of group analysis. They define the parameters of group analytic thinking as incorporating the political and social environment with all its components, like power differentials and class boundaries, as well as the basic human conditions as a social animal, without which we would never have survived as a species. We need each other, we are dependent on each other and in order to function, we need organisations and structures for groups and communities, regions and countries, as well as globally. These, in turn, imply power differentials.

The following three chapters define the political and the social in slightly different ways, reflecting each the particular view and also vision of their authors. All three papers focus on the importance of the political and the social sphere and the impact these had on the work and lives of their authors. They describe how power relationships and the awareness of, for instance, class differences pervaded not just their personal upbringing but also affected their professional choices and career developments, as well as their ways of thinking and now of working with their groups.

Diane Rogan-Sofer introduces the notion that the environment we grow up in is affecting our perception of the world and our position in it to a considerate and lasting degree. She introduces the rarely used Freudian concept of disavowal, since she considers that this mechanism has a significant impact on past and present power dynamics. Understanding the consequences of disavowal, she argues, sheds light on the contemporary political context and dynamics of power. It highlights the pain and hurt that underlies political value shifts towards more extreme and radical positions as a way of defending against loss of self, powerlessness and shame.

Eugene Clerkin takes up Foulkes' notion of the social as a colossal force that permeates us to the core. He makes a passionate plea for the necessity to recognise the dialectical nature of the individual as social, and the social as political, something that is not always recognised in the field of group

DOI: 10.4324/9781003310358-6

analysis, let alone in the domain of mental health in general. The individual and society as a whole are often unaware, even unconscious of these social forces and are defending against recognising how strongly we are modelled by them. He asserts that the social is always in relationship with and never distinct from how a society is run and structured, which is political. Political power relationships, where some have more power than others to shape and structure their lives, always make society antagonistic and unequal.

Sue Einhorn reveals in this lecture, originally given at the Israeli Institute of Group Analysis and again three years later to the Group Analytic Training in St. Petersburg, the influence that her historical and political family background had on her confidence and self-worth but also on her educational development and her later work life. Her background together with the consciousness of class and a strong feminist attitude have contributed to her capacity of being in the exceptional position to describe the strange phenomenon of being a group analyst.

Chapter 4

The political and the personal

Diane Rogan-Sofer

The current global context and the effects on the individual and the group

We are living in and through turbulent times. Global political alliances are changing, and global economic markets are developing ever further. Un-checked capitalism and neo-liberalism, far right political movements and religious fundamentalism are on the increase. Terrorism and wars and their aftermath have given rise to increasing mass migration.

This unsettled global context has enormous consequences. Relocation of industries in pursuit of profit has left areas within the UK with high unemployment. Unemployment causes stress and anxiety for individuals and families. Changing needs of the market-place have left many without the necessary skills to actively participate in the economy. Young people from working-class families are put off applying for universities because of the introduction of tuition fees. Immigration, always a feature of the UK, has recently become once again a political tool, with which to provoke fear of the outsider through political propaganda. We have been able to witness this in the often obvious, but also subliminal messages in the lead up to the 2016 referendum. Hostility in regard to difference and a longing for the em-pire of the past have led, as sociologist and academic Helen Davis wrote, "a falling back on a mythical history" (Davis, 2004). And as academic Barnor Hesse said "the so-called homogeneity of British culture has been massively overstated" (Hesse, 2000). Consequentially, social divisions are growing.

Mental health illness, particularly in the young, is increasing. The cur-rent culture of over-diagnosis and over-medication is indicative of a system which blames and shames individuals for problems, which they must resolve individually. We know though that the problem is in the group as a whole, not just the individual and their interpersonal relationships. The problem is out there in the social, in society, the social unconscious, described by S.H. Foulkes as 'colossal forces' in all of us (Foulkes, 1964, p. 258). We all carry a responsibility to address the social, political and economic conditions,

DOI: 10.4324/9781003310358-7

which are making increasing numbers of people unwell and affecting future generations.

Politics is about state craft, the practice of government and its administration. It is also used to describe relationships within social structures, from work-place office politics to personal domestic relationships. Simplified, it describes relationships to power. Eugene Clerkin, in his essay 'In the Realm of the Political', says:

> ...the social is always in relationship to the political and is therefore never devoid of the political forces that permeate the individual. ...The political as a power relationship, where some have more power to structure society and their lives than others, makes society antagonistic and unequal....
>
> (Clerkin, Chapter 5, this volume)

We have a duty of care to examine how the internalisation of political power structures might influence us and how they manifest in the conscious and unconscious dynamics of our groups.

What has been done and what needs to be done

In the current political situation, it seems essential that we ask some probing questions. Is working as a group analyst or as a psychotherapist a political action? Was the decision to train as a group analyst a political one? What is group analysis in relation to society? Does group analysis promote a sense of citizenship?

These are pertinent questions. Promoting a dialogue about them while exploring the connections and differences between the political and the personal, more questions may emerge. I want to begin by talking about the issue that concerns and moves me the most, which is social class. My personal experiences regarding class have formed my identity and informed my decision to train as a group analyst. They continue to influence how I work. They have influenced my values and have formed my political and personal identity.

The issue of class constitutes a meaningful focus for me in regard to two infinitely large subjects, the political and the personal. Class as we know is a huge sociological area and recently has re-emerged in public discourse after having been marginalised for a long time. Everyone has their own experiences and ideas about class. I want to keep especially the following aspects in mind, since I feel they are the most relevant when thinking about class:

- The emotional impact of inequality: the sense of hopelessness people experience when they cannot compete in the way the market currently demands; the hurt they experience when they or other persons are overlooked.

- The public shaming of individuals or social groups: shame as a psychological tool used for manipulation to maintain the status quo.
- Widening schisms: increasing splits and separation between those who have and those who have not; splits leading to loss of empathy and the loss of the willingness to engage with difference. These splits undermine the necessary conditions for normal human altruism to flourish.

Working class and psychoanalysis

A lot has been said about the missing voices of the working classes in Sigmund Freud's writings and about their roles in society. This oversight has been written about by a number of clinicians and academics working in the field, most recently by Joanna Ryan in *Class and Psychoanalysis* (Ryan, 2017). Referring to one of her examples, nurses and nannies, the surrogate mothers of the children of the upper classes were not mentioned by Freud. They were considered either invisible or were debased in such a comprehensive way that their existence was wiped out of any theory, apart from being objects of sexual fantasies. The biological mothers, often emotionally distant and often physically absent figures in Freud's patients' lives, take nevertheless centre stage in Freud's theory of development.

Recognition or appreciation of the nanny's attachment to their adoptive children and theirs to her and their shared intimacy seems to have been an impossibility. Only fear and envy of her role existed and was frequently followed by a denial of the trauma of separation and loss, when she, the 'intruder' to the family, finally left. The notion of 'ungrievable lives' suggested by the feminist academic and psychoanalyst Judith Butler is relevant here. In 'Precarious Life' (Butler, 2004), she explores whose lives are grievable and whose lives are not and discusses why in her view this is so.

A great deal has been done since Freud's time to promote changes in therapeutic practice. There is for instance an attempt to actively engage working-class clients, for example in specialist women's services. Nevertheless, the disavowal of class, when "conscious awareness of painful realities is rejected" leads inevitably to "a loss of moral valence", as described by psychoanalyst Hinshelwood (2008). Hinshelwood's description, as well as Professor Stephen Frosh writing in *Sitegeist* (Frosh, 2009), refers to the focus in psychoanalysis on the biopolitics of identity, gender, sexuality and race whilst forgetting class consciousness. Frosh argues that shame is a dynamic at the heart of the psychoanalytic profession for a number of reasons, primarily that love has become a commodity that is bought and sold through exchange of money within a capitalist system, and shame is linked to anxiety within psychoanalysis of contamination by poverty, getting too close to economic need.

In order to survive as a profession, psychoanalysis needs people who suffer. The 'betrayal' Frosh talks about is linked to the shame and the fear of exposure of one's investment in not confronting class issues by not acknowledging the "damage one does by virtue of being in a position of dominance, and to hear that others' needs (which Psychotherapy and psychoanalysis are supposed to ameliorate) are produced by their closeness to necessity" (Frosh, 2009, p. 12).

The neglect of class, he argues, might have something to do with the profession's desire to remain amongst the 'salubrious professions' (Frosh, 2009). This 'occluded' memory, that is the forgetting of class roots, constitutes however part of the foundation matrix of psychoanalysis and therefore group analysis.

The social impact of inarticulation

Talking about class is problematic. Interestingly enough, this applies to anyone and also to someone coming from a privileged background. Ryan (2017) talks about the difficulty of symbolising and articulating thoughts and feelings about class, when – as is the case in society – social positioning forms an important part of identity and personality.

Reflecting on the difficulties of articulating thoughts about class, these ideas help to understand that this may be linked to being from a particular social class, whose subjectivity is disavowed. This may well be coupled with a contemporary class position of privilege, and this may leave the individual feeling self-conscious and unhelpfully aware of their social position. The effect is to compromise symbolisation and the freedom to articulate thoughts and thinking.

Inarticulation, the repression of pain and the negation of pain by others can lead to an accumulation of intolerable rage, fuelled by an underlay of narcissistic wounds. This, in turn, can lead to an explosion of destructivity, in words and actions. The group analyst Dennis Brown (2006) captured these processes in his book *Resonance and Reciprocity*, when he reflected on the aggressive actions of football fans, following the defeat of the Scotland team playing Peru in 1978 World Cup in Argentina:

> We do not know their individual stories, inner worlds or social circumstances, but from their appearance it looked as though they were indeed the bottom of the social pile for whom the only activity to restore self-esteem in, say, a Glasgow slum, would be to turn the tables on the rest of society by joining the National Front, or making a fantastic journey to South America in search of gold – not in El Dorado, but in a vision of themselves as clean-limbed conquerors of the world. The tragedy was to see their free speech reduced to the spat-out words 'rubbish' and 'scum'.
>
> (Brown, 2006, p. 78)

This may be a somewhat dated example, but it captures well the processes we could all witness in more recent political contexts. In my view, the recent British referendum result uncovered an enormous degree of damaged self-esteem, brought about by political and economic forces, which were blind to the hurt done to large parts of the British population in the pursuit of profits and global economic success and power rather than social good. The referendum result may well be a major incidence of the consequences of political negation and the disavowal of social responsibility. Free speech has become reduced in this case to a protest vote – driven by ill-informed ideas and lies, fuelling fantasies of an idealised notion of empire, where life was simpler, and people seemed to be more similar. The long-term consequences of the referendum, still unknown and not looking too good, will without doubt make exactly the very same people continue to suffer the most. The referendum has created a schism between individuals, families, communities, counties and countries within the UK, which feels extremely difficult to repair.

Inarticulation and communication in group analysis

Both these examples, the historical loss of memory in psychoanalysis, as well the recent protest vote of the referendum, are examples for the results of a kind of speechlessness and disempowerment. According to Foulkes, we emerge as individuals from a matrix, which is in fact a complex web of communications. In his theory, communication has priority at many levels, non-verbal as well as verbal. Dennis Brown (2006) noted that words can 'block and foster communication'. When talking about politics, he asked the pertinent question, if 'free association' was the same as 'free speech'? He concludes that sometimes honesty and truth have to be modified in order for the individual to be accepted by his or her group. Do our therapeutic groups provide the opportunity for group members to hide until they feel ready to openly speak with their own authentic voice? Or do the groups foster conformity, or do they do both?

It is hard to communicate freely and authentically when a whole class system of uncommunicated injustice and pain is part of the picture or even constitutes the context. Under those circumstances, it is a struggle to be polite and can take a lot of energy. Real, that is, authentic, communication may even be dangerous, especially when real divisions and differences emerge. Seamus Heaney (1975) makes that clear in his poem 'Whatever You Say, Say Nothing', where he describes the impossibility of talking openly about politics in Northern Ireland in recent history but also points out that indirect communication went on anyway. Heaney's poem describes the need for conscious recognition of the 'other', as well as an unspoken recognition of religious affiliation and class, and how dangerous talking about any of this can be in times of civil unrest.

The contemporary novel *Milkman* by Anna Burns (2018), set during the troubles, describes the main character's capacity to compartmentalise her inner world, necessary in order to survive the fear of madness brought about by living in a context of constant threat, inconsistency, contradiction and paranoia. When the character looks back from the future at her eighteen-year-old self, she describes not only the inarticulation of her then thoughts, but her mind's capacity to protect itself by not allowing the thinking of the thought in the first place. No names are used throughout the novel, too dangerous to be known, so the hidden inner world is reflected in the hidden identities of the characters. When there can only be a right or a wrong, as is the case in binary thinking and psychotic states, any known identity might have very dangerous consequences.

The personal context

Major transitions in childhood give anchors to memories, which inform our sense of self. This changes over time, it is kinetic, a slowly changing materiality. If you were born, for instance, somewhere in the Northeast of England, like Newcastle Upon Tyne, you end up feeling a Northerner, even after having been living in London for over twenty years. There are many strata also in the white working classes even in the North, and the colour of a collar noticed in one's formative years can remain a defining feature. A lower-middle-class 'white-collar' family home may stand in contrasts with the steel town, the place of this family's home. It is a place divided by class, with blue-collar workers in the steel works and white workers in the civil service or more middle class professions. There are also dividing religious affiliation, Catholic, Protestant and Methodist. After closure of the steel works in 1980, unemployment rose to 38%, three times the national average. Very little was done at the time by the government responsible for this decision to relieve the hardships of the working-class communities. The communities of the steel towns were forgotten, disavowed. Forty years on, the area still has not recovered, one of many areas in the UK that fell victim to globalisation.

The impact of economic pressure and unemployment on every family caused stress, anxiety and frustration and ricocheted through the community. It was impossible not to see the inequalities and their impact on the lives of people. Which side of the tracks you lived on made a real difference to your life. Experiences like these imprint early on an awareness of class differences and class struggles, and people often develop a burning desire to distance themselves from those struggles of poverty and economic need and to have a different life. Some manage to get away and may become the first in the family to go on to higher education.

College then becomes a further education in the dynamics of power and class. University towns often have ghettos for their black and Asian community, with white working classes and students in separate areas. Consequently, students have very little opportunity to meet anyone with a different skin tone or significantly different culture. Despite these borders and barriers, white working-class students and the black and ethnically mixed community are clearly bound together by economic marginality, as referred to by the academic, writer and activist Stuart Hall in John Akomfrah's documentary film 'The Stuart Hall Project', *The Unfinished Conversations* (Akomfrah, 2012).

The political context

Antonio Gramsci (1891–1937) argued that "different social, political, economic and ideological contradictions came together to form distinctive historical moments, which he called 'conjunctures'" (Gramsci quoted by Stuart Hall, 1987). During the rise of a neoliberal political agenda, the Thatcherite years went along with the notion that "There is no such thing as society" (Thatcher, 1987). It was a period of increasing contrasts. 'Yuppies', striving for wealth, and encouraged to be ruthless in the pursuit of profit, could be found in opposition to social activists, who challenged the state through protest marches. Creative flourishing in the arts and music and a desire for a new political order emerged, based on serious concerns about the planet, a growing ecology movement, interfaith dialogue, multiculturalism and third wave feminism. This moment constituted such a 'conjuncture'.

Jessica Loudis in 'The New Republic' (Loudis, 2017) wrote that Hall argued that the political left had not been able to counter-balance Thatcher's political move to normalise, and make 'common sense', neoliberal ideology. He felt that

> Thatcher did not succeed by tricking voters, but rather by constructing a worldview that mapped onto their real lives and problems (if not their class identities) and advancing policies that reflected those concerns

and takes this as a reminder that

> interests are not given but always have to be politically and ideologically constructed.
>
> (Hall cited by Loudis, 2017)

What was missing was a counter claim, that contrary to 'no such thing as society', the working classes excelled at creating societies and communities. These societies knew for the most part how to support and care for each other, to manage problems and understood mutual dependence and reciprocity. They also knew how to come together in political activity to present a strong counterforce to unchecked capitalism.

Once again we find ourselves at a 'conjuncture' and it would appear the political left still does not understand that ideology is influenced and formed by the political messages communicated through media, which reach into and actually resonate with peoples' real lived lives.

Power, collusion and the care system

I had finished college and needed a job at the time and my degree opened doors. My first job was as a volunteer in an inner city mental health drop-in service for young adults. This led to a paid position with Social Services in a residential unit for children who had experienced sexual abuse. These children had no boundaries, theirs having been both physically and emotionally transgressed. They were hyper vigilant, desperate for affection and deeply vulnerable. Their chaotic unpredictable behaviour caused high levels of anxiety for the staff, who, with the exception of a few, managed this anxiety with authoritarian regimes. Challenging behaviours were seen as tests to personal authority, not as communications of profound disturbance. Witnessing this, I felt silenced by the abuse of power, which profoundly affected my sense of integrity. At the time I did not know Menzies Lyth's (1960) seminal work on organisational dynamics to help me understand and articulate the disturbance I felt. Perhaps I also did not fully comprehend the shame I felt leaving these children. I had a choice, they did not.

Continuing training involved moving to another city and a placement in a residential Therapeutic Community, helping young people who were self-harming. These youngsters were outside of their families and the mainstream education system, often isolated, self-destructive and difficult to engage. It was difficult not to be affected and feel overwhelmed by their experience of being out of place in both class and culture, struggling to articulate their rage and pain within themselves and in relationships with others.

After qualifying, I worked in an NHS medium secure unit. Here patients were mostly from poor white, black and Asian working-class communities. Case histories were littered with experiences of loss and damage, severance of early parental relationships, often through immigration motivated by economic need and poverty. There was a huge lack of education and social isolation. Weekly case meetings were deeply troubling. It seemed as if the power relationships between classes in society were concentrated here in an intense focal point.

Spaces for societies' location for shame

I have found that also the majority of group members in training groups and in my own group analytic groups had personal histories of growing up in poverty, materially and/or emotionally. Places like children's homes, community mental health services, hospitals for the treatment of serious mental health illness, HM prison services, but also university counselling services and other such organisations, are all places that hold and contain a disowned aspect of society. These places, I suggest, are socially organised spaces for the containment of pain, humiliation and shame.

Power, authority and psychotherapy

My decision to train in group analysis, rather than embarking on a dyadic training, was based on my personal experiences, which informed my values and subsequent political affiliations. I believe we all have our political and personal reasons to train in either group analysis or individual psychotherapy or both. Group analysis offers a democratic model, founded in Foulkes' premise that the conductor is as much a part of the group as everyone else. Since everyone else in the group is also learning to be as much an analyst as is the conductor, this allows groups to develop an identity based on equality and shared responsibility. I believe this is the reason why power relationships can be acknowledged in group analysis and engaged with. There is more safety in a group and more transparency, since there are witnesses and abuses of power hopefully do not go on unseen. Foulkes said:

> Relatedness, seen as taking place within a basic all-embracing group matrix, is the corner stone of our working theory.

> (Foulkes and Anthony, 1957, p. 236)

While group analytic factors and group phenomena are crucial in understanding the deep communication in groups, I would agree with Foulkes that group analysis' most important contribution is the group's potential to develop 'relatedness', to build bridges between the members and to develop empathy and understanding of each other.

But have we as Frosh (2009) said 'domesticated the unconscious'? Psychoanalysis has a history of taking the 'wrong path' and 'going astray' (Laplanche, 1999, p. 67). Have we chosen ease-of-mind rather than the discomfort of facing class conflicts within our profession? We are as vulnerable to bureaucratising conformist pressure as is any other profession. Perhaps dropping class from our agendas is evidence of a resistance to the actual 'critical tradition' of psychoanalysis.

Political change, Donald Trump, power and politics

For the most part, I have felt to be part of a democratic system, which is moving forward towards a more socially aware, empathic and humane society. But I am wondering, if I have not recognised until now how privileged a view this was, and I also wonder if I have been engaged in an unconscious disavowal. Perhaps instead, democracy has been undermined by unchecked complex market forces and blinkered 'political narratives', leaving us all vulnerable to the spread of extreme ideologies, far right agendas and radicalisation. I am concerned about the impact extreme inequality has on dividing and divided communities, causing schisms and making it harder to cross cultural boundaries and engage with class difference.

Looking back from our current political context, we might conclude that neoliberal policies and effects in the past, which prioritised profit and power above all other concerns, were a mild forerunner to what has led us now to a widening of the gap in wealth, health and economic and educational opportunities, complicated by the rapid rise of technology, which has led to the mechanisation of industry predicted by Karl Marx over a century ago (Marx, 1974).

These reductive developments have led to increases in fragmentation of working-class communities and weakening of social cohesion, leaving large numbers of global citizens disavowed and disarmed, unable to come together to form a powerful challenge to an all-for-profit model of global capitalism, and understandably enraged.

The widening of the gap in values and ideology of political parties causes real concerns of annihilation. Jessica Benjamin in her opening lecture at the Psychotherapy NOW Conference in November 2018 (Benjamin, 2018) described how she understood the current social schisms in the United States. She described as their basis the 'The Wolf Position' or the view that 'Only One Can Live Versus More Than One Can Live'. Benjamin talked about how the idea of 'Only one can live' is embedded in the United States social system and its Calvinist religious belief system, which divide the deserving from the undeserving.

Benjamin then described the complex processes of projective identification, with the help of which the struggle to be able to live is being played out in the United States through erasing the 'other', because of the fear that otherwise 'you' will be erased. The rights and dignity of the other seem to threaten the self. The identification with powerful people, for example, Donald Trump, allows people an unconscious process of denial of shame, guilt and vulnerability, which would ensue if the harm done to others was acknowledged. Benjamin (2018) stated that these unconscious processes have led to the strengthening of the current far right movement. The task ahead is to find ways of symbolising recognition of these processes for all.

Altruism and the foundation matrix

This means for me that we must ask what group analysis can offer to help mitigate these forces, which will continue to undermine principles of equality and human dignity, if left unchecked.

During his time at the Frankfurt School, Foulkes was influenced by ideas from human biology and neurology about the existence of altruism. In his lecture at King's college, the political commentator George Monbiot (2018) challenged neoliberal ideas of basic human selfishness with the counter-argument that we, the human species, are designed to be altruistic. Foulkes recognised that it was the context, which was crucial in influencing the balance between selfishness and altruism.

Dennis Brown (2006) optimistically talked about an emergence of a new consensus of awareness, stirred by globalisation of economics, communication technology and the internet. This consensus, he wrote, recognises mutual concerns and rights linked to responsibilities towards each other, to our own and to other communities and to the planet. It could be said that he is talking here about citizenship, but I wonder, if his viewpoint was too optimistic, given events at the present point in time. However, what he reminds us of is that ideas of belonging through relationships are essential to human evolution and progress. It is mutual concern, which involves responsibility to and for others as well as citizenship, through which relationships and happiness are found. These ideas are at the very core of group analysis and contain within them the potential to lessen the currently existing schisms both internally and externally.

Our groups are spaces where we communicate with the help of dialogue and where we can develop mutual concern and empathy, where we can create a sense of community by learning that belonging and being given help by the group also comes with a greater understanding of the group members' responsibility to each other. This makes the group a 'third space'. As Brown and Pedder (1987) said, groups are places where members can over time develop

> ... a capacity for concern for others in the process of defining and developing oneself.
>
> (Brown and Pedder, 1987)

Group analytic groups are places where individual needs and the care for others have space to co-exist. However, they are also places where class divisions are rife, the conductor included. To resist our own shame, shame linked to fear of loss of status, and moving closer to dependence and need by denying the existence of real economic matters in clinical practice and to interpret power differences only as an intra-psychic dynamic, silences the group and leaves painful class histories and here-and-now realities unarticulated.

Conclusion

As group analysts, we need to comprehend more fully how our position in the power hierarchy of the psychoanalytic profession may have burdened us with a feeling of inferiority, leaving us to be too quiet, withdrawn, inarticulate and enraged. Group analysis is made by, and develops, through the people who constitute and benefit from being in our groups. It is eminently important that we reflect on our internalised power structures and ask ourselves how our community, whilst a membership organisation and a form of representative democracy, may be able to change to give more space for the voices of not just a privileged powerful few, but everyone, to be clearly heard.

A final question in my mind is if we do need to be more visible in the public arena as a profession. Many colleagues have taken up the challenge to take group analysis to a wider world, to international conferences or meetings of GASI or EGATIN for instance. Can group analysis also closer to home be more outspoken and outward looking and engage with the political arena in society, as well as with the personal in clinical practice? This is not a new idea, but it seems to be a continual stumbling block. What needs to change in order for group analysis to be more outward looking? Do we need to practice more what we preach? Do we need to go further in acknowledging our unconscious shame and our own vulnerability, our needs and our fears of slipping further down the social class system?

Chapter 5

In the realm of the political

Eugene Clerkin

Introduction

I chose this topic from my experience of being in a therapy group as part of the training to become a group analyst. I began to think of difficulties in talking about my politics in group therapy. This led me to question if politics was considered not to belong to the scope of group therapy, or even seen as irrelevant to personal relationships and the psychological domain. In my opinion, this omits an important area of life from exploration and creates problems for the theory of the social in group analysis. Foulkes' notion of the social, which he saw as a 'colossal force' (Foulkes, 1964, p. 52), would be limited only to the much narrower interpersonal social sphere.

I am arguing that the social is always in relationship to the political and never devoid of political forces that permeate the individual to the core. How group analysis interprets the social leads me to focus on the impact of the political on the individual that can be occluded from therapy into a more limited 'psychologised' form of understanding. It is argued that this has consequences in the clinical setting, where fundamental aspects of the patient's communication or 'total situation' (Foulkes, 1948, p. 15) can be prevented from reaching dialogue in the group.

The term 'political' as an adjective refers to governmental or public administration forces of the state. However, the word 'politics' is used far more widely to describe relationships within institutional structures, from work situations or office politics to governmental structures and ideologies in general. The term 'politics' I understand therefore as describing relationships to structures ranging from the highest authority, for instance national or international powers, to the domestic and local relationships of everyday life. Everyday life experience within its private social context is itself located within greater contexts or structures that form what Elias (1978) described as the figuration. This is the nexus between people and the unit of analysis within the figuration out of which the 'I' can emerge, as one cannot imagine the 'I' without 'he' or a 'she', a 'we', 'you' (singular and plural) or 'they' (Elias, 1978, p. 123).

DOI: 10.4324/9781003310358-8

Foulkes' (1964) theory of the social, a force that is compelling and which permeates each and every one of us to the core, has not been represented in the literature as the socio-political force that it is. With his use of the word 'colossal' in connection with the social, he wants us to recognise the immense power and impact of the social domain. In Foulkes' view, the social determined the individual as much as Freud's notion of the id, as can be seen from the following quote:

> Moreover, the individual is as much compelled and modelled by these colossal forces as by his own id and defends himself as strongly against their recognition without being aware of it, but in quite different ways and modes.
>
> (Foulkes, 1964, p. 52)

The implications of this are enormous. Foulkes tells us that the forces of the social are equal to the dynamics of the individual's unconscious by introducing the notion of social forces as compelling. The notion that the individual is unaware, even unconscious of these powerful social forces and does not want to know about them, is extremely important in this context. Similar to our defences against the recognition of the id, we are also defending against recognising the way we are compelled and modelled by the social. However, we do this in quite different ways and modes. I think this requires us to examine these different, necessarily wider and varied modes of defence and look at what our patients might show us in that respect.

In order to do so, I will now present a clinical example to show some of the complexities of the personal within political realms and vice versa of how the political manifests in the realm of the therapy group.

Clinical example

Pauline is a 39 years old white working-class woman. Her parents worked in a local factory until the premature death of her father from a lung disease caused by a reaction to industrial dust. Pauline spent several years caring for him until he died. During that time, she fought his former employer for compensation but failed. Following this she trained as a primary school teacher, but increasing bureaucracy led her to leave. Her feelings of failure were strong and left her with thoughts of having 'nothing left'.

During her first few weeks in the group, Pauline could not really explain to herself or the group why she was there. She felt as she did at work that the group was mundane and irrelevant. It seemed to her that the majority of the talk was about difficulties in personal relationships that she increasingly felt frustrated about. This heightened her anxiety about feeling able to tell the group about her rage and her political views. For example, she had strong feelings about the country going into a war with Iraq but thought that a topic like this might not be perceived to be personal. She therefore had not yet told the group that she was planning on joining an 'anti-war' march and being an activist, as she was not sure that it would be seen as group business.

A month into her attendance, there had been several security scares nearby that made some people late for the group. Clare, a mother, talked about police presence 'these days in the streets' and how terrible it was that 'this is necessary now'. Pauline timidly said that she thought police presence was there to make people more scared. Clare exclaimed 'What...?!' Pauline said in a nervous tone that she thought that this was to prevent people from protesting or voicing their opinions, rather it was to silence them. There was then some silence in the group, after which Tom began to talk about how quiet his home was now, following his divorce, and that he also finally realised how much had not been said between himself and his ex-wife. Then Jim asked: "We don't talk about things like politics here?"

Pauline looked anxious and scared but was silent. Many months later she could tell us how anxious she was then so as not to stand out. She was clearly in two minds about actually engaging in talking as this might create, in her mind, 'too much' conflict and she would be blamed for it.

It took a few more weeks before she could tell the group how her father died, and how angry and powerless she felt that he had not been compensated for the industrial disease that killed him. Clare responded by saying that she thought Pauline was really talking about her 'own' agonies and isolation. Pauline said that this frustrated her and that other group members often talked about how others' needs reflected their own, and that this attitude left her feeling that whatever she tried to say would get misinterpreted.

Discussion

What is going to enable Pauline to engage further with the group and talk about how she felt? In the scenario described above, group members are emphasising Pauline's unconscious feelings and fears. This could be a denial of or resistance to social facts (Hopper, 2003a) since it puts the accent on internal reality. For Pauline, her rage with the powerful employer – a social structure – has become linked to her bereavement, but her grieving cannot really start until the dialogue in the group can include her feelings about the betrayal of her father. At this point in time, Pauline's feelings get re-characterised and re-interpreted by the group only in a psychologised form of understanding.

Six months later

Jim is a middle-class professional white gay man. He talks about his optimism for society's progress in its increasing acceptance of gay people and how much this has improved his life. Pauline says that this isn't the same for the underclass and the unemployed. She continues that his politics are focused only on his identity and that this blinds him, which leads to an argument and Pauline's feeling that the group is ganging up on her. She is told, in turn, that she is continually blaming society in a way that allows her to avoid her own 'real' pain, and that this blinds her too.

Discussion

Pauline resists knowing something about herself, and the group resists knowing her. The temperature in the group is raised when she attempts to communicate her desperation. What is it about her anger and bereft feelings that have not yet reached the group? I wonder if this is because there has not been enough communication and exchange about the nature of each group member's own particular social matrix. Have I as the group analyst not yet been able to bring or weave in the social as an unconscious phenomenon into the language of the group? Pauline as a group member also perpetuates this dynamic, often by not speaking. Locked in these antagonisms no-one sees the other's perspective.

How can the group analyst intervene here? Pauline is in a dilemma. She experiences the group as distant and offering her little flexibility to find and shape her own space within it. I am also in a dilemma. I am not sure how to intervene in a way that does not occlude Pauline's social and political matrix but would also take her personal isolation and bereft feelings into account. The group appears to offer no prospect for an encounter that would engage group members in a greater exchange.

Eighteen months later

In July 2005, Pauline had been in the group for over two years. Following the London suicide bombings, the concomitant tension finally brings the group to boiling point. At the beginning of the session, there is silence. Pauline looks scared and remains tight lipped. Then Clare comments how awful it is with so many people killed and maimed.

"Why can't they talk?" asks Jim.

There are expressions of outrage and terrible anxiety.

"This country isn't safe anymore", says another group member.

Pauline remains silent and seems to me even slightly disengaged. Jim mentions her silence. Pauline, referring to the British state and its involvement in Iraq and Afghanistan, then says:

"They had it coming".

Clare is outraged and begins to shout at Pauline, telling her that she is an irresponsible person 'with all her politics'. Feelings overspill.

Into this atmosphere of utter fear and awkward tension, I say after some minutes:

"Perhaps it's too unsafe to talk about violence and fear, as both feel present".

Jim says that they both are very close.

I ask: "Can we talk about what feels so close?"

Pauline says: "The violence today was in reaction to the State's violence".

Clare, in a calmer tone, but still annoyed, says: "So you react with violence to violence".

This led on to talking about causes of violence. Tom asked both women, if they had ever been violent and this then led to further exchange. The group is beginning to grapple with the question, where violence is located, within an individual or between people? Foulkes (1948, p. 127) emphasised that any disturbance, even that with deep roots inside the individual, affects the group as a whole.

Discussion

The impulse towards splitting and projection of violence is apparent in the above example. The question here is what needs attending to that will allow the group members to connect with each other when the divisions seem so entrenched. My attempt to name both fear and violence appears to hold or contain the group members' feelings to some extent. It made it more bearable to stay with the tension and the current reality of the group's dynamic.

Later in the same session, Clare tells us that her daughter has been unwell for some days. She says, how protective it makes her feel and how scared it made her in thinking of her own vulnerability. I say that perhaps everyone in the group feels vulnerable about violence and their own violent feelings are spilling over here. The group becomes quiet and more sombre, which I understood as moving into a more 'work group' phase (Bion, 1961).

Two months later

The group begins with Clare telling us about her child, who is still unwell and now being investigated for a rare bone disease that is possibly life threatening. Pauline is clearly affected by this and asks Clare about the illness. Clare tells her that it is rare and that treatment is particularly expensive. Jim tells us that he is reminded of Pauline's fathers' death. A theme of fear and loss is present. Pauline and Clare stare at each other, clearly with feelings, and tears are shed. All the group members feel moved. There is a loosening of tension. Feelings emerge that enhance exchange.

Three weeks later Clare tells Pauline that her fears for her daughter made her think of Pauline. She had felt such anger as well as fear, when a physician told her that if her daughter had a particular type of bone disease, the treatment might not be available on the NHS. It made Clare both angry and terrified at the prospect.

Discussion

When the group members could begin to link with each other through feelings of loss, which had previously been resisted, it became possible to start piecing together what Bion described as a matrix of loss and gain, a bargaining, or the beginnings of working through to the 'work group' phase (Bion, 1961).

This had been impossible before the group could meet Pauline's gripping resistance to grieving for her dead father. Her identification with Clare's situation in regard to her child arose out of a deep sense of resonance. For Pauline, the material conditions that contributed to her father's death were real and not an avoidance of personal responsibility, just as real as her feelings. Clare, in turn, had been closed to Pauline's 'there and then' (Hopper, 2003a) personal and social situation, until she found herself in a similar situation. There was now an engagement with each other. In the group an atmosphere developed, which allowed room to attend to both women's wider social matrix.

The psycho-social and the political

I will return to my original question of how do we as group analysts work in our groups with the social and interpret it in its wider context? How do we use our understanding of this in our groups and our lives?

In order to begin to answer this, it will be necessary to unpick what is meant by the social. The word social might easily be confused with the word society. In Collins Dictionary (1999), social is described as that of living, or preferring to live in a community, rather than alone. It is related to human society, to experience and personal interactions, and to the purpose of promoting companionship and communal activities. Society on the other hand refers to the totality of social relations among organised groups and a system of human organisations that generate distinctive cultural patterns (ibid). From these definitions, we could say that the term social is a process or description of people together, either through desire, within relationship, or when placed or living alongside each other.

Mead's Social Psychology (Reck, 1964) places the self within a social structure and sees the two as inextricably linked. Burkitt (1991), who draws on Mead's work, shows us how we respond to ourselves as objects of our own subjectivity. This means that the 'me' aspect comes about through the internalisation of how others relate to me. Individuals respond or relate to themselves as others relate to them. This illustrates Elias' (1978) figuration as a basis to understand the social as made up of the individuals embedded in a community in close proximity.

Foulkes tells us that we are permeated to the core by the social. I find his term 'permeation' helpful and I want to use it to try to explain why I argue that the social is political in the following analogy. Water, for instance, cannot flow upwards – or permeate – without a power-source driving it. But it can nevertheless be pumped in any direction by a greater force. The point I want to make is that permeation is not a 'free flow', but it involves a force. The force involved is an analogy for those who make decisions or those who have the power to organise the flow of water – or organise society.

Force and power

How do force and power as constituents of the social get expressed as societal phenomena? I am arguing that both are in relationship to each other, whenever force is a driving momentum or an expression of power. Force in the physical sense can move and deform matter. When it is exerted or used against a person or a thing that resists, it has the power to form, shape and thus determine the shape or the movement of the object it is forcing.

When we translate this idea of force to the realm of human relations, we can see ourselves as being deeply formed by others and forming each other in a social matrix beyond the merely personal contact. To go to work, for instance, is seen as a natural activity which is not normally questioned, as there is no alternative to this in a society based on money as a medium of exchange for daily essentials. However, we need to or are 'forced' to earn our living. I contend that it is this 'forcing' of our individual activities that therefore makes the social political. Though each of us having certain degrees of power as described by Foucault (1992), some people, through ambition, privilege or social class, are placed in positions where they are able to use power over others. This then creates an uneven power dynamic, since some do not have the same power as others to determine their life in a way they might want to. However, we are all of us part and parcel of that structuring process and its various figurations.

The social is therefore an inter-relational structure that is dominant in our lives and dominated by structures through the organising of society that makes it political, as power is used in the organising of it. It is more than a personal or interactional force but is always constrained or enabled by dominant forces and powers which are beyond individual control. Power exerted by the political is shaped through ideology, which is usually out of personal scope, but nevertheless a dominant force.

Ideology can be thought of as a body of ideas that reflects the beliefs and interests of a particular community, a nation or a political system. I found myself wondering, why ideologies are so often hidden and obscure. Maybe as Szasz (1973) stated, there is a clear limit to 'man's' freedom – namely the freedom of other 'men'. This is another way of describing the constraining aspect of the social. It brings ideology into everyday experience and this is a particular aspect of Hopper's (2003a) work on the social unconscious. I cannot explore Hopper's work here further, but these ideas have immense consequences for group analysis. Firstly, they show us that ideology is omni-present, like a current in the river, the wind in the air, or the force of gravity. It is always present and can be experienced by its immediacy in the atmos-phere. It is something that cannot be stepped out of.

Discussion

How do we as group analysts stay in touch and work with the political matrix, bearing in mind the psyche and the social – as political? Classical psychoanalysis theorises the individual instincts that configure our life's journey, as arising from within the individual psyche. Marxism on the other hand asserts that it is material forces, especially economic production that shapes our destiny. Jacoby (1975), a social historian, in his critique of con-formist psychology, for instance, suggests that psychoanalysis and historical materialism are both fractured pieces in and of a fractured society. I agree with him that attempts to 'harmonise' a synthesis of Marxism and Psycho-analysis presuppose a society without the antagonisms that are in fact its essence, as this avoids the tension within that dialectic that is required to work with the social as political.

I hope that these thoughts draw attention to the risks and dangers of reducing politics to psychological notions and interpretations on the one hand, and of explaining psychic suffering in terms of the political and ne-glecting the subjective factor on the other hand. I want to point out that in order to avoid these dangers, it becomes necessary to maintain the dialec-tical tension that allows for the articulation of both individual emotional states and of how these stand in relationship to the societal and politi-cal matrix. It is the central point of this chapter to assert that we need to find ways to pursue two different logics simultaneously in our work with groups. We need to develop the ability to retain the tension between the interpretations of Marx and Freud, and those between the individual and the political.

This means we need to think about our own ideological presuppositions and question them. How can we allow discussion of our own 'unequal' social position as the group conductor to enter into the conversation in and of our groups? As we have seen, the social is more than a fence di-viding or a chain linking people, delineating different social positions or places of power, but something immense, with constituents that effect, drive and coerce our activities every day in our lives. If we can consider how the structuring and organising of power is done and carried out, and by whom, we introduce power relationships into the matrix. In this pro-cess, we as group conductors play a part, no matter how constrained or enabled we are.

The clinical example shows how hard it was for the group to find ways to see the political aspect also in its personal dimension, because it appeared that the personal only referred to close relationships. The dialectical nature of the relationship between the two aspects of the personal and the social and political needed exploring, so that it could become possible for the specifically personal feelings of loss and grief to be attended to in the group. In other words, it was necessary to explore the political first in order to get to the personal.

Conclusion

In conclusion, I want to summarise that I have argued that there has been a tendency to understand the social with too strong a bias towards an interpersonal perspective, rather than with a view to the wider social arena, so that the consequences of the political matrix can also enter the dialogue. Where this is avoided in the group, consciously or unconsciously, there exists the risk of an exclusion of the political, hence of the political aspect of the personal. In order to avoid this, it is essential to pursue the dialectical tension and the bi-focal vision between the individual and the political matrix.

The purpose of this chapter is to help us consider how to make the importance of the social and the political conscious for group therapy with the inclusion of communication about it in the group. A lack of awareness of this can lead to a narrowed and psychologised form of understanding of the patient's social matrix. Foulkes thought of communication not only as a process but also as a communion, an existing communal network, where through the work of the group, a matrix can grow and develop, which, in turn, increases the capacity of the group to embrace and grapple with those more complex issues, that is the dynamic matrix (Foulkes, 1975).

Chapter 6

The strange phenomenon of being a group analyst

Sue Einhorn

Introduction

At a time in Europe when psychoanalytic perspectives are under attack and finding the space for reflective work is increasingly difficult, I have found myself wondering how and why I became a psychotherapist and why was I drawn to group analysis in particular. I will look at the wish to understand and to belong that struggles with fears of annihilation. This struggle is not just with psychoanalytic thought, but also with issues such as climate change, economic collapse, the refugee crisis and religious conflict, in other words, an increasing level of acute existential anxiety. Perhaps the key word is struggle, because when I was young and a political activist, the struggle was to contribute to a world more just. Now, the struggle is to understand the complexities or impossibilities of being human and how to manage ourselves in our personal lives, let alone influencing the world around us.

It seems to me that the constant struggle is to maintain the integrity of what to do in a hostile, judgmental world with attacks on allowing a sufficiently reflective space, where the 'mute symptom', the unknown, can be discovered and given a voice (Foulkes, 1964, p. 68). I believe we need to be able to 'feel with our minds', what I call 'an emotional mind'. This is the essence of analytic therapy of all modes, and this is what I have tried to teach (here in Russia), but it is being attacked, because in a time of anxiety such therapy cannot be tolerated. I am interested in why we, you and I, choose to become therapists and so I am using this opportunity to explore my personal journey and hope it will stimulate connections for you. After all, you are the future!

A space to think

Some years ago, in response to Gerhard Wilke's Foulkes' lecture (Einhorn, 2007), I spoke about the freedom a reflective space can offer, when, whatever happened, happened somewhere else. 'Here' is safe enough to think, whereas 'there' is where it happened. Usually, we locate the 'there' as having

DOI: 10.4324/9781003310358-9

happened in childhood and we return to that strange place as adults, at a particular point in time, because the past intrudes or enhances the present. For instance, Gerhard Wilke could think more clearly about his experiences in Germany through making his life in England (Wilke, 2007). Perhaps this also links to the 'Father' of Group Analysis – S. H. Foulkes – who developed his ideas in the UK in his thirties having been born in Germany in 1898. He came to the UK in 1933 when he was thirty-five years old being invited by Ernest Jones.

He trained as a psychoanalyst in Vienna but joined the British Psychoanalytic Society in London and moved to Exeter in 1939. The move away from the psychoanalytic community did give him some freedom, and perhaps we owe the development of Group Analysis to his move to Devon, where he was free to bring his learning from Germany together with his experiences in the UK. I was reminded of his situation by the thoughts that I wanted to explore, when asked to give a paper here in Moscow. I feel freer here to express my thoughts as I look across to the UK but also back through time. Why, as I reflect on my forty years of work, do I continue to find myself absorbed in other peoples' struggles and deprivations?

Learning to be a group analyst

This particular thought occurred to me as I was sitting in one of my therapy groups some weeks ago. It was the last session for a very long-standing group member. He had been in the group for nine years, and he was talking about the journey he had shared with us. As he and we remembered, I found myself thinking, why do we do this? Why did he, and why did I? After a few years of therapy, he decided to train as a group analyst and, like most of our trainees, he had to learn how to be a conductor in a hospital or prison settings, where patients are suicidal, borderline and very disturbed. He managed well and was well supervised by the clinic where he was practising.

However, there he was a trainee and being assessed. As you all know, patients like this get under our skin and perhaps even more so in groups. What trainees bring to their own therapy group is their pain, their depression, the preverbal traumas that they, and also many of their patients, had experienced. One of my trainees insisted that what she needed from our group was for her to remain mute. Sometimes she would cry, and sometimes she would tell us about her envy of others, but, for months at a time, it would be impossible to reach her.

Both she and the man I mentioned before had to struggle with being unable to think, being possessed by rage and losses that they could not make better with words. At times they would disappear from the group, leaving us to manage their absence, while they struggled with feeling lost and abandoned. As inexperienced trainees, they had been plunged in the deep end and the fragmented, raging, hurting parts of themselves were endlessly triggered by the people in their training group, for whom they had responsibility. The question 'Would their group survive throughout the training?' could be translated into whether they would personally survive.

Survival

Both psychoanalysis and group analysis developed during periods of war. The context of war has often been a creative time, because, I think, fear of survival arouses questions about the very nature of being human. Hope resides in the need to try and understand, to hold onto the mind when all around is reaction and fear. Foulkes, as we know, trained in Germany when terrible things were brewing but held on to the duality of human beings. Morris Nitsun (1996) explores Foulkes' lack of attention to aggression and hatred, but perhaps, like for my parents, knowing that aggression was around, meant also to Foulkes surviving it. Interestingly, for people like Foulkes', for my parents and perhaps for many of you in this room, survival is about finding one's mind, finding the capacity to think, to search for meaning and to bear to reflect on the experiences that have been so disturbing. Perhaps only when survival is secure, can the whole picture, including human cruelty and hatred, be reintroduced into the present. How do you create a safe reflective space when worried about your survival? Our trainees have their therapy group, in order for them to have a secure, steady space to which some of this very unsafe emotional work could be brought, as part of their therapy.

I do love groups and have been in them all my life in different ways, but I became a group analyst because I also hate groups. The competition for space, feelings of envy, jealousy and rivalry or feeling overlooked or incompetent, and above all, the ever-present fear of being shamed make groups in many ways harder than the hidden and secret pair in one-to-one therapy. How painful all this is. Recently one of my colleagues asked if I had noticed how many group analysts had stopped conducting groups. He is very experienced but said that his groups give him more sleepless nights than all his other work. I agreed. Why then do we do this to ourselves? Why become a group analyst?

As we know, choosing to be a psychotherapist often includes needs for reparation, both towards the inner family that was felt to hurt and, also, as a need to explore the transmitted traumas unprocessed by one's family of origin. So, let me begin there.

The Ten Commandments

My parents were communists through a very deep sense of wanting to fight for a fairer society. Their commitment to communism may have been a very different one compared to that of people, who have actually lived under a communist regime. They were educated by the communist party in Britain, my father having left school at thirteen and my mother at fourteen. They were East London Jews and brought me up after the Second World War with the following 'Ten Commandments' and I will link these family commandments to the tenets of group analysis later. Perhaps these commandments are similar for everybody who wishes to become a group analyst. You could also make your own list after this lecture.

1 Remember that although the world is not a fair place, human beings will be good in a fair world.
2 A real human being is one who contributes to society.
3 Ordinary people should be given a voice, as they know what really matters.
4 Thou shalt seek to be informed. Not knowing is no excuse.
5 Don't trust non-Jews/don't trust anyone outside the family.
6 Thou shalt not dwell on the past. Thou shalt despise the casualties of the past within the family.
7 Your children are the purpose. Jews defeat the enemy by the regeneration of the family. We children were symbolic – standing for a defeat of fascism, a defeat of the anti-Semite and we were the purpose of the struggle.
8 Thou shalt make every effort to assimilate with the locals and avoid a Jewish Ghetto Mentality.
9 Education is the real church. Education includes culture. The love of music, literature and art transcends the basic struggle to survive in a hostile world.
10 Never get into debt and always make sure there is enough for the emergencies that will be bound to happen.

The story of my family's escape from Russia was never told. The place from which they came was never mentioned and the costs to the family in terms of death and madness were suppressed. Madness was a family secret and there were many family secrets.

The story of Foulkes' move to the UK has also not been properly told, it was a particularly British Jewish experience. This is a complex issue, because Foulkes understood the importance of history especially in relation to his colleague, the sociologist Norbert Elias (1994). But Foulkes somehow managed to separate that from his own personal history, probably because he had family that perished in the Holocaust.

For me as well, you trainees are the purpose, like children, as you are the next generation of group analysts. For my parents, it was safer to 'pass' as non-Jews, so I was called Susan Janet. It meant that we would not be penalised by anti-Semitism and would not be unable to join the communist party.

I wonder what is sacrificed by needing to belong. When arriving in Britain, Siegmund Heinrich Foulkes changed his surname from Fuchs, which means 'fox', to Foulkes, but was called Michael Foulkes by friends and family, although he would call himself S. H. Foulkes in his writing.

Was my choice of group analysis rather than psychoanalysis linked to a wish not to be assimilated? It is not the conventional psychotherapy path. The 'Ten Commandments' show the extent to which my relationship with my immediate family was instilled with history, with rules of distrust, anxiety and insecurity, with trying to belong, but not really belonging. All these ideas were essentially secular. Being Jewish had nothing to do with God, but everything to do with feeling excluded or at risk and it was the potential within the human being that needed to be nourished and cultivated by the right sort of social context. Somehow the right society would transcend the past, an unbearable past that could not be spoken about.

To explain this a bit more, Commandment 1 meant that the right social context was a 'safe' group, which would then conform to Foulkes' Basic law of Group Dynamics (see also Tucker, Chapter 14 Normative Authority, this volume). This states that

> the deepest reason why patients...can reinforce each other's normal reactions and wear down and correct each other's neurotic reactions is that...collectively they constitute the very norm from which, individually, they deviate.
>
> (Foulkes, 1948, p. 29)

Social activism and psychotherapy

In my twenties, I turned my back on Jewish roots and decided to contribute to society by becoming a community activist and a feminist. I was determined that ordinary people should have a voice (Commandment 3). This entailed committees and meetings and protest rallies. Twenty-four hours was not enough. At the same time, I was part of a consciousness-raising group to explore how to liberate myself from the social oppression of being a woman.

We need a story to hold us together, but I was very unclear about what my story was, and what belonged to my parents and the commandments I had internalised. By my thirties, I realised that however hard we worked to reorganise society – and at the time I genuinely believed that a social revolution was possible – we also needed to understand our inner worlds. For example, we may believe that women and men were politically equal, but I could see that feminists and political activists were not living these ideals privately at home.

The view of the Women's Movement that 'the personal is political' emphasises that it is only by understanding how the external world 'penetrates to the core' that society could become a fairer place. Through the Women's Movement, I understood that the isolated mind and the individualism of psychoanalysis did not include 'the political'. In contrast, in group therapy, the human need for connection and relationship (The need to belong, Commandment 2) is seen as essential and it includes an understanding of the unconscious.

I was still politically motivated but, desperate to put myself into words, found a psychoanalyst. I lay down on the couch and he said nothing. I felt abandoned, ignored and as lost as I had been when I was taken into care as a child with my sister for about a year. I was two and a half and whatever language I had was lost. This was not explored in my analysis, because I was desperate to please him, so that he would give me some attention, but none of this was understood. He fell asleep and I felt a failure. So I became a group analyst, very much in the spirit of my family's ten commandments.

Trust and the group

Groups are extremely potent places for exploring the nature of trust and respect. I want to digress a moment into trust – you may remember Commandment 5, which was really suggesting that I should not trust non-Jews or anyone outside the family. But how could I really belong to any group or community without being able to trust?

Group members trust us, when we suggest a particular form of therapy, but this is trust in us as a therapist or analyst, the transference to our role. This kind of trust may be more often submission, a submission arising from the desperation that has made the person seek therapy in the first place. This is very different to learning to trust the group or the group conductor with emotions or a history that feel unsafe. It is not unusual for group members in a session to withhold, fantasise or even, on occasions, lie. I think we need the group to be able to develop clear judgement about who is safe, whom to tell and when to risk trust.

When Foulksian group analysts talk about 'trusting' the group, I think they are describing a mature group, where members are interested not only in their own problems but also in those of the other members and in developing the sort of relationships within the group through which members can help each other. As Caroline Garland writes in 'Taking the non-problem Seriously' (Garland, 1982), the therapeutic quality of the group develops, when the relationships with group members include beginning to care for and wanting to engage with each other as siblings or friends. Then members begin to trust other members with the difficult aspects of their history and are able to tell it to people who want to know. The therapy is really in the development of relationships that nourish, both within the therapy group, but also outside in members' personal lives.

This is a political thought, as well as a Foulksian thought, because it implies a more democratic form of therapy. My family's Commandment 3 certainly agrees with Foulkes that the group is the therapist, and that members can often be more influential than the conductor, since the conductor's job is to observe the boundaries and keep the group safe.

What does it mean to keep a group 'safe'? In a safe group, there is space to reflect on oneself and to think about the other members. I have written about this before (Einhorn, 2018). It is a place where the difficult, often unsafe, because painful and shaming, relationships of the past are re-lived through the present relationships in the group. But this time they can be thought about, and their meaning understood. Safety resides not only in the group conductor but also in the regularity of the group and sufficient confidence in the conductor's authority to help the group to manage conflict or attend to 'unspoken' themes. All this is not the conductor's responsibility alone.

The need for groups

Foulkes was part of a generation that venerated psychoanalysis, but in group analysis, he developed a method that also included other aspects, like, for instance, Kurt Goldstein's approach to neuroscience, Elias' sociology and history, Moreno's systemic thought, and Freud's teachings (Pines, 1982). Group analysis has always been inclusive of other disciplines and has been relational from the beginning. As Nitsun shows in the 'Anti-Group' (Nitsun, 1996) this presented Foulkes with a dilemma, as he also wanted to be accepted as a psychoanalyst. If we consider that man is relationship-seeking from the beginning, and that this is the primary instinct, then it makes sense that we may also want acceptance from people or groups that do not understand us. This creates a problem as groups are counter cultural.

The UK has developed as an individualistic culture, where there is shame in needing others, but little shame in being exposed on reality TV shows. It seems there is a secret longing to have as much individual attention as possible, but this is shameful to acknowledge. One of the attractions of belonging to a diagnostic category may well be that this gives permission to have 'counselling'. Not the whole person needs attention, only just the bit that needs mending, like bereavement, over-eating, psychosis and so on. That is one reason why people find it strange when we suggest a group, when people come into therapy. "Why would I want to share you?" a client asked. When I point out that ordinary people can help each other, if they feel safe and heard, clients say: "Why come to a therapist then?"

Often people come into therapy because they are preoccupied with feelings of shame, envy, jealousy or emptiness. These feelings make relationships difficult. When group analysts suggest that these are exactly the areas where group therapy can help, it may take a lot of courage or submission – often described as trust, although there has not been any time to develop real trust – or quite a lot of desperation to agree to group therapy. Once in a group, the feelings of shame and envy painfully emerge, together with a re-awakened sense of deprivation. So much that goes on in group members' lives cannot be expressed, as the space in the group is shared and time is limited. People have to learn how to get the group's attention, what is useful for them to express, and often have to tolerate waiting yet another week before they can talk, if they can still remember what they wanted to say by then. No wonder groups erupt from time to time. Sharing with siblings can be rewarding, but is it rewarding enough to make up for that familiar feeling of deprivation, of never getting enough, of not being heard, of not being found?

Fundamental to therapy is Foulkes' idea of the symptom being mute and needing translation into language (Foulkes, 1964, p. 68). The language can be ordinary words or metaphors, but they need to be heard and worked with, so that a patient feels understood and found. So many of our patients feel lost or abandoned. As a man in one of my groups said the other day: "It's only here that I have found my despair and only here that it feels safe". So maybe groups do work.

The intensity of groups – or the ongoing theatre of the group and in the group – can evoke the life-force, a sense of vitality, in the patients' world, where even hatred can be better than numbness or emptiness. It is at such times that the conductor may well have sleepless nights, as we are being asked to contain symptoms that as yet have found no expression but are being experienced and wish to be found.

The feeling mind

What I want to emphasise is that above all, group members and patients need our minds. Whatever our intuition or capacity to recognise feelings in others and in ourselves, we need to be able to feel with our minds or develop an 'emotional mind', if we are to be of use to our groups (Commandment 2). I think most theories of therapy describe ways to recover our minds and help us to think with our emotions. It is precisely that capacity that can be so easily attacked by groups, and not only groups of course. Resonance can be toxic as well as harmonious, and that is when we have sleepless nights.

The current debate in group analysis seems to centre around instinct theory versus intersubjectivity. Are we driven by forces essential to the nature of the human animal or does being properly human depend on our capacity to learn how to relate so that an inner 'real' self can blossom? I have to confess I find both perspectives persuasive, depending on the state of my groups at a particular moment in time. Should I learn MBT, CBT, DBT or other techniques for working with certain categories of people? I find all these techniques fascinating and useful when learning about them, and I find myself thinking of particular patients or group members when attending such courses. However, I regard all these theories and techniques as 'pencil sharpening'. To be able to feel with my mind or think emotionally in the service of my group members or my patients, I need ideas and words to translate what they are saying, feeling or projecting, that my mind can engage with and at the same time use as a separating function between us. I need an intact mind to remain a therapist or group conductor and be of service to my patients.

'A Real Human Being is one who contributes to society' (Commandment 2) and I understand this to be the therapist's contribution. To do this, our theories and techniques offer us particular ways of understanding the 'reflective space' essential to our brand of group analysis, but this should never impede on the value of simply staying with not knowing. Our emotional minds may struggle hard to remain with confusion, sometimes even with panic, but I believe this struggle is the real value of our reflective space in groups. It is a shared, sometimes unknown space, where we wait for understanding to emerge, often through metaphors or dreams, but eventually, over time, in words. For example, a woman who had been expelled from her childhood country during war, periodically re-entered a shocked fugue state in the group, so that she could be found and led back again into the current safe world of her group. At first, we were all – including her – very disturbed by this, but later, over time, as this was understood, we were able several times to reach her and help, until the behaviour finally receded.

Conclusion

My decision to become a group analyst arose at a more unconscious level, out of the wish to repair internalised destructive feelings due to a legacy from my parents, who, in turn, also had not been able to emotionally process historical experiences transmitted to them. The secrets that could only be felt had created fear, but I wanted to understand and so I tried to be informed. This was the result of Commandment 4 – Thou shalt seek to be informed. Not knowing is no excuse.

My closing thought is, of course, the question of age and getting older. How do I evaluate whether I have been useful? I find groups challenging and see them as privileged places, but I am also aware that I love being a therapist, which means working with people in distress. Freud says we are pleasure seeking, so I wonder what pleasure I am gaining from this work? Has being a group analyst helped me to grow and, more crucially, has it made me ready to face my own mortality? After all this will be my next developmental challenge. The survival of group analysis will be decided by the outside world, but as psychological thinking is under attack and we become more accountable for what we do, I am aware that I need to evaluate myself as well. Am I competent to evaluate myself or is it part of your job, as the next generation, to evaluate your teachers, including me?

Am I out of date? What role does the internet play within what I call 're-flective space' and 'emotional mind'? I am happy to learn from other forms of therapy and I want group analysts to be accountable, politically, as well as for reasons of integrity, to group members and other agencies who use our methods of work. However, it is not easy work and the intense demands of retaining an intact emotional mind in the service of our work needs to be acknowledged. I do believe that group analysis can offer a reflective space, where we can continue to try and understand not just the patients we work with or the group members who attend our groups but also use it to struggle with trying to understand the world around us, even if this world cannot always wait for our slow, process-driven, revealing form of therapy.

Why are you a Group Analyst?

Part 3

Diversity and difference

Introduction

Diversity and difference are two further basic concepts in group analytical thinking. Difference and diversity arouse curiosity and can also provoke fear. They make us take notice and if the anxiety is not too great, they make us think. Then we learn through difference. It is one of the preconditions for any group analytic group that it is conceived as a 'stranger' group. Members in a group analytic group are not supposed to know each other or have any contact outside the group, since this guarantees confidentiality, which is important for any therapeutic endeavour. In addition, 'strangeness' means novelty; it arouses interest and can also introduce an element of friction and tension into the group. Having to deal with newness and difference requires an attitude of open-mindedness, which, in turn, fosters tolerance, both important aspects of maturity.

The first two chapters in this part ask if and how group analysis as a method can be applied in non-Western settings. Can group analysis accommodate and manage aspects of cultural diversity? Both these chapters present work with non-English-speaking groups with people from completely different cultures and this raises important questions. One of the groups took place in the UK, another in Africa. The work in Africa had to consider the effect of differences of race and skin colour, and also explores aspects of working with interpreters as part of group analysis.

The next chapter explores the notion of the social unconscious, an important concept of group analysis that expands the notion of a personal unconscious known from psychoanalysis. Specific differences between group members, regarding gender, sexuality, class, colour, ethnicity, language, culture, nationality or other social factors can provide an entry point to working with the social unconscious and may signal the need for analysis of the underlying social conditions. The conductor needs to be aware that this work may be essential to help the group deal with specific conflicts which may otherwise be seen as personal and remain unresolved.

DOI: 10.4324/9781003310358-10

The last chapter in Part 3 describes working with a very particular difference, that is, between mothers and babies. Here the central role of communication in group analysis is demonstrated. The variety of different ways of communicating is so much more than just verbal, and this is here shown at work.

Seda Sengun reports on her work with a Turkish-speaking women's group, investigating the applicability of 'Western' thought and practice in a different cultural context and assesses how this affects the development of a group and its members. Of Turkish origin herself and with Turkish as her mother tongue, she explores the emotional impact of the shared cultural background on the conductor and states the necessity for developing a cultural sensitivity not only to openly question the impact of culture but also to challenge what at times is presented as a cultural norm.

Justin Phipps describes his involvement in a group analytic training course in Rwanda, East Africa, where interpreters were present in the groups. Rwanda's extreme trauma and socio-cultural norms have shaped what can be articulated verbally. The use of open communication, as suggested in group analysis, is seen as ambiguous, and indirect communication and proverbs are often used instead. While also questioning the applicability of group analysis under these circumstances, the chapter demonstrates how group analysis played a part in gaining new insight and understandings for the participants.

Sylvia Hutchinson focusses in the next paper on the role of the social unconscious and suggests that it needs more attention in therapy groups. The chapter is an edited version of a talk given in Warsaw in 2004 to celebrate the tenth anniversary of the founding of the Warsaw Institute of Group Analysis. It concentrates on the social forces, which are shaping our attitudes, often based on unconscious elements derived from our social and cultural environments. Subgroup formations, which form around specific differences between group members, like for instance gender, sexuality, class and colour, can provide an entry point to working with the social unconscious in groups.

Sheila Ritchie describes work with mothers and babies in an NHS Perinatal Mental Health Service. In this work, both parties gain the experience of being in a social setting with peers. Both, mothers 'and' babies, are involved in the therapeutic work as equally contributing partners despite the babies' lack of language. This highlights the central importance of any kind of communication, not exclusively verbal communication, in group analysis.

Chapter 7

A Turkish-speaking women's group and the cultural considerations in everyday group analysis

Seda Sengun

Culture, social unconscious and group therapy

There are many different definitions of culture. Winnicott (1953) defined it as the inherited tradition, as something that is in the common pool of humanity, to which individuals and groups of people may contribute, and from which we may all draw if we have somewhere to put what we find. Le Roy (1994) wrote that culture on one hand contains the undifferentiated and unified aspects of the individual psyche and on the other hand that it promotes the structuralisation of the psyche through its introduction into a series of symbolic orders. However, my favourite definition comes from the field of anthropology. In anthropological terms, culture is simply, "The system of shared beliefs, values, customs, behaviours, and artefacts that the members of a society use to cope with their world and with one another" (Anthropology course notes, University of Manitoba, Canada, May 2019).

Culture is in most parts unconscious and only becomes visible when the person is in a different cultural context. It is internalised from the other members of one's culture, including parental figures. As such, it includes at least the family, class and national cultures. It permeates each person and the groups they belong to, and therefore it impacts on all human behaviour, thought and belief system from religious rituals to sexual practices.

Culture is very much a part of the social unconscious. Hopper (1996), writing about the social unconscious in clinical work, described it as the existence and constraints of social, cultural and communicational arrangements of which people are unaware. Unaware in so far, as these arrangements are not perceived (not 'known'), and if perceived, not acknowledged ('denied'), and if acknowledged, not taking as problematic ('given') and if taken as problematic, not considered with an optimal degree of detachment and objectivity. Indeed, frequently the impact of culture on the psyche is not known or denied or accepted as given and not considered with an optimal degree of objectivity. As a result, a considerable part of the person (or the group) gets missed or overlooked.

DOI: 10.4324/9781003310358-11

Culture has affected how psychoanalysis and group psychotherapy is practised in different countries. The Brazilian psychoanalyst Figueira (1991) proposed that there are 'national psychoanalyses' resulting from the interaction of universal psychoanalysis with the particular cognitive, emotional and ethical structures of a given culture. Along the same lines, van Schoor (1997) argued that the American ethos of individualism impacted upon group psychotherapy, promoting an ideology of the private and autonomous individual. This is, of course, very different from the Foulksian approach which sees the person as a part of the social network, 'a nodal point'. Foulkes (1948) wrote that

> the individual is not only dependent on the material conditions, for instance economic or climatic, of his surrounding world and on the community, the group in which he lives, whose claims are transmitted to him through the parents or parental figures but is literally permeated by them. He is part of a social network, a little nodal point as it were in this network and can only artificially be considered in isolation, like a fish out of water.
>
> (Foulkes, 1948, pp. 14–15)

There are many articles written in the 1980s and 1990s, mostly on transcultural counselling and a few on group therapy, but the interest in culture and psychotherapy has slowly declined, particularly in the past decade.

One set of articles, which seem to be mainly from the United States or affiliated professionals, is mostly about how the 'Western' originated group therapy (or psychotherapy in general) cannot be applied as it is to so-called non-Western clients and groups; or it is not as effective, due to the cultural differences. For example, Berman and Weinberg (1998, quoted in Weinberg, 2003, p. 262) wrote that "cultural norms might prevent groups from developing towards advanced stages, such as intimacy". Chen et al. (2008) wrote:

> Cultural diversity expands the multiple perspectives that are already available in the group but also limits within-group communication, presenting an increased risk for misunderstanding and conflict.
>
> (Chen et al., 2008, p. 1264)

They went even further and cited Clark et al. (2000) as

> cultural heterogeneity in group work, …has been found to be associated with decreased communication, performance, and satisfaction as well as higher conflict and turnover.
>
> (Chen et al., 2008, p. 1264)

On the other hand, group analysts trained in the Foulksian approach wrote about culture either in the context of the transcultural group analysis workshops (Brown, 1992a, 1992b) or in the context of working with so-called non-Western groups in clinical settings (Devan, 2001; Sengun, 1997, 2001, 2003) and as part of a group analytic training (Beck, 2015; Lorentzen et al., 2006). Their conclusions are very different. They agree that while the cultural norms impact on the group processes and can slow them down, they do not prevent groups from developing towards advanced stages, such as intimacy or maturity. In fact, in everyday group analysis, we try to provide in our groups as much diversity as possible.

My experience of working with Turkish patients and groups also confirms this finding. In a response to Haim Weinberg's paper (Weinberg, 2003) on groups from different cultures and his conviction that "Cultural norms might prevent groups from developing towards advanced stages, such as intimacy" (Weinberg, 2003, p. 262), I wrote elsewhere (Sengun, 2003) that, in my experience, this was not the case at all. I gave a vignette from my Turkish Speaking Women's Group to illustrate this. At the time of writing, the group had been running for approximately two and a half years and I had left the reader with some questions about the long-term future of this group. Now, many years later, having continued running the group until the end of its tenth year, I can follow it up.

In this chapter, I will examine how cultural issues, including my own, might have impacted on this group and whether the group was able to go through the usual process and whether it reached the advanced stages. I will give a brief description of the group and report on the progress of its members. However, I will begin by looking at some of the writings from the two different perspectives outlined above.

Group therapy with ethnic populations using non-Foulksian approach

I am concerned about the difference between my understanding of group therapy, including group analysis, and the work reported in some of the articles. Should every therapeutic activity, which takes place in a group setting, be called group therapy? Or could doing so and publishing results from this mislead the reader in terms of what group therapy is and its outcomes? That is what happened when I read Chen et al. (2008) and their citation above. I was rather taken aback that the multicultural therapy groups caused so much difficulty and felt compelled to find the original paper they referred to. It turned out that the article was nothing to do with therapeutic groups at all, in fact the authors are from a College of Business Administration. They clearly state at the very beginning that "we [authors] develop a model of interpretive resolution process…in newly formed diverse decision-making work groups". To apply findings from such a group to therapeutic groups is grossly misleading. I also found that the actual wording in Clark et al. refers to 'demographic heterogeneity' not 'Cultural heterogeneity', a difference worth noting and another misleading point.

Kinzie et al. (1988) described a one-year experience of 'group therapy' for people from Southeast Asia who were treated in a psychiatric programme for Indochinese refugees. They thought that the cultural factors involving communication styles, respect for authority and traditional social relationships greatly influenced the group process. They reported that therapeutic activity occurring in a group setting, employing varying techniques and sharing of practical information were the most acceptable medium by all the groups in the program. Psychological issues of loss, cultural conflicts, and persistent discussion of somatic symptoms were voiced throughout the activities. However, the formal group psychotherapy was only 'periodically' useful in some groups. They concluded that flexibility, meeting concrete needs, keeping a bicultural focus and maintaining the individual therapy sessions contributed to the acceptance by the patient. Here the authors make a distinction between therapeutic activity groups and 'formal group psychotherapy' in which specific interactional and dynamic issues are examined.

Coming back to more familiar psychotherapy groups with culturally diverse membership, Tsui and Schultz (1988) presented a framework that was generated by clinical experiences with Asian clients in predominantly Caucasian therapy groups in a psychiatric setting. Their focus was on the impact of differing perceptions of power, authority, interpersonal boundaries and family process on group dynamics. Meanwhile, Yamaguchi (1986) and Kotani (1999) described the impact of culture on Japanese groups. Yamaguchi wrote that the respect and reserve given to authority figures as well as subtle and indirect communication style make group processes less straightforward than in the West. Kotani stated that "a regular nondirective process group would fail in Japan", because the members would feel threatened by the push to express their individuality.

The group analytic approach to cultural diversity

Lorentzen et al. (2006) from the Institute of Group Analysis in Norway wrote about their experiences in setting up a group analytic training in Lithuania for the Baltic countries. They discussed the impact of the cultural differences on the large group processes and on setting up the training. Although both programmes reached mature stages, the original Norwegian programme took about two years to mature, whereas in the Baltics, it took three to four years. Beck (2015) reported about an experiential group process over two years as part of a psychodynamic psychotherapy training in Shanghai. He asked: "Does the application of the group analytic approach in such a different culture with such a different foundation matrix make sense?" (Beck, 2015). After giving a touching account of the group and its processes, he concluded that he was

> very impressed as to how much could change in the course of only 56 sessions despite the fact of the very different foundation matrix in the

Chinese cultural context. This experience seems to prove that it makes sense to apply the group analytic approach even in such a different culture.

(Beck, 2015, p. 156)

Dr Sathya Devan, who is a Singaporean clinician, but trained in group analysis in London, conducted a slow-open, multiracial psychotherapy group in English in Singapore over an eight-year period. Most of the patients had improved symptoms as well as improved interpersonal relationships and ability at work. Devan (2001) identified several unique, culture-specific group processes concerning authority, individuation and intimacy. He wrote quite openly about his struggle of having been trained in the West and trying to apply his learning to his own community in Singapore and the difficulties in the transference/countertransference, with which I fully concur. He wrote that despite the pressure to be directive, observing Western supervisors, who were more permissive, enabled him to become more non-directive in his style.

Nigerian Okeke Azu-Okeke wrote from the perspective of being a trainee and a patient in a group analytic group. He comes from the Igbo tribe who believe in the power of the ancestors and practice ancestor-worshipping. Also, in Igbo culture, there is a taboo on discussing family matters with the strangers. Azu-Okeke wrote (1993):

My experience as a group analysand involved a process of examining some of my personal values and prejudices .... Some of the responses from my group felt like deliberate malicious attacks on these values. At the same time, it felt as if the group was envious of what I had to offer them from my culture. The hallmark of this experience was that it made examination and evaluation of my traditional culture obligatory. To be a member of a strangers' group (my analytic group) would have been unthinkable were it not for my face-saving pretence that my training requirements made this obligatory. But as time went on I became aware that I was doing what I had secretly needed to do and desired to do if it were not for the hindering taboos that preserved the traditional norms.

(Azu-Okeke, 1993, p. 266)

Azu-Okeke concluded that the process of group analytic training enabled him to overcome some of his stereotypical views and to gain more understanding of his 'self' as an individual member of his collective traditional society.

The Turkish Speaking Women's Group and its members

During my group analytic training, I ran several homogeneous Turkish women's groups ranging from three months to a year. Even in such a short time, the groups were useful in making the women aware that there were different realities than the ones they experienced and change was a possibility. They wanted more therapy. Encouraged by these groups, I set up a new slow-open group at the Women's Therapy Centre in London once I finished my training.

My first mistake with my Turkish group was to initially name it the 'Turkish Women's Group'. During the assessments, I realised that there was no such thing as 'Turkish women', since each referral I received was different from the previous. One woman was from a Kurdish background, the next one was from another Turkish ethnic minority on the Black Sea cost; one had come to the UK as she was married off by her family, the next one had emigrated to work so she could send money home, and so forth. And of course, there I was, with my own history, my own reasons for immigration, my class and my own family culture which was very different from any of the group members. This was the first time I really understood that 'culture is not monolithic'. Hence, the name for the group became 'Turkish Speaking Women's Group', not counting the accents!

The original five women in the group were in their thirties, from Turkish, Kurdish and Laz (another Turkish ethnicity) backgrounds. They were all married and had children. Two were economic migrants, one was a political refugee, and two had arrived through marriage.

The histories included abuse as a child or neglect and deprivation and often required having to look after siblings. One was mistreated as a girl at home by both parents, only allowed to go to primary school and married off at a very young age. The two economic refugees had to leave their young children with their own mothers and struggled to bond when the children joined them some years later. Several carried a racial trauma.

Two members presented with severe anxiety and panic attacks, somatic symptoms and occasional pseudo-psychotic episodes during which they would hallucinate. These intensified during the breaks or when the therapeutic process got extra difficult. Both were on an antidepressant and a small dose of antipsychotic medication. All others, except for one, were on antidepressants as they had anxiety and depression which were often expressed through somatisation.

Two new members joined the group after two and a half years. They were both very different from the original women in the group, but at opposite ends to each other. One was an older woman from a village. She was an illiterate and highly dependent woman, a stereotype of her generation and background. She was unable to recognise or express any feelings for the first two years she was in the group and took no responsibility for her own actions. Yet, she had been able to convince me to take her into the group.

In contrast, the other woman was from an urban and educated family. Both parents were professionals, but nevertheless, it was a severely dysfunctional family. She was a university graduate and well read. She presented with personality problems and loved shocking the group with her stories of misbehaviour. Not only was she different from all the other group members in her language, accent, dress code and activities, but she also was the only member who sounded and looked like me, because of the proximity of our cultural backgrounds. The group struggled with both of these women for a long time, and so did I.

Guilt and shame were regular themes in the group, as well as victimhood and rage. To begin with, the members very much saw themselves as victims and insisted that that had nothing to do with their family dynamics. However, a few years later, they began to change. A woman who was particularly rigid in her thoughts and quite resistant to my comments, exclaimed one day as the group was discussing victims and perpetrators: "Oh my God! When the children were young and made me angry, I used to lock them in a cupboard. That means I am the perpetrator, aren't I?"

I was shocked to hear this and I still remember it vividly. At the time, I could not tell whether I was shocked because I had thought 'locking children in a cupboard' was only a figure of speech, or because I was hearing such a significant insight after such a resistance to therapy. In any case, the more she explored how she might have perpetrated against her children and her husband or others, the less victim she felt. Some months later, she told the group how she had sat her children down and apologised to them. She said in tears that nobody had ever apologised to her for what they had done to her and as much as she felt guilty for harming her children, she also felt proud that she could ultimately be different to her own parents. I also felt proud of her.

Another woman struggled with her relationship with her daughter when she became a teenager in a very different culture than the one she had grown up in herself. Throughout the life of the group, she presented to the group as a severely controlling mother figure who wanted to live her life through her daughter. However, she appreciated the group very much and therefore was slowly able to hear the protests of the other women in the group: leave her alone! Through defending the daughter, other women in the group gradually found their voices. The group worked together through the mother's envy of her daughter. She eventually let go of her control and allowed her daughter to go to university in another city. Her daughter's 'freedom' was celebrated by the group members as if it was their own.

The older woman eventually managed to receive therapy and the group became more and more her favourite activity. She underwent an amazing transformation and the group was gripped by her genuine sense of humour. She enrolled in an adult literacy class and also learned to use her matriarchal power to help other women in her extended family. She became the epitome of change and hope for the group.

Overall, the members managed to process their traumatic experiences, mourned their losses and, eventually, gained a real confidence. A couple of them attended English classes and got part time jobs.

The first member to leave the group, having had barely missed a session in eight years, gave six months of notice. Her leaving provided the group with an opportunity to work with separation. She was followed by another member a year after.

Difficulties in the ongoing management of the group

This group was one of the most difficult groups I run in over twenty years of practice, yet it was the most memorable, rewarding and educating group. It was already a difficult group because of the homogeneous nature of it, the high level of disturbance it contained, and the heavy use of projective mechanisms members used, as they were not able to express feelings in any other way. On top, I had to deal with my own transference, identifications and prejudices almost in every session. For the first couple of years, I felt as if I was surrounded by five mothers of mine! Then, with the new member joining, who was close to my own cultural background, I had to watch myself vigilantly in order not to get caught up in identification with her, but also with the group's tendency to treat her as a co-therapist which made the group easier for me.

To begin with, it is normal for any group to be dependent on the therapist. However, in this group, dependency was not only much stronger but also took much longer to resolve. In addition to the power the conductor naturally holds, the cultural tendency to relinquish all responsibility to a higher authority meant that I was the only one who could make them better. I felt the heavy burden on my shoulders and felt frustration and resentment. In hindsight and after many years of experience, it is easy to see the projective mechanisms at work, but at the time, I had to rely on weekly supervision quite heavily to create a space in my mind and between myself and the group. I wrote in 2003:

> In my Turkish speaking women's group whenever I made interpretations about the separation process and the boundaries of the self, members either ignored me or got annoyed. At times I became convinced that I was running this group in a completely wrong fashion and it was no use to them.
>
> (Sengun, 2003, p. 270)

Another dynamic I used to find difficult in the group was the endless physical complaints and the competition as to who was the most ill member. I was very familiar with psychiatric patients who presented with bodily symptoms back in Turkey. In fact, this was just ordinary in that cultural context and time. However, after living for two decades in the UK and training here, it felt unbearable to me. These silent demands on me, expressing both idealisation and aggression left me feeling depleted after each session.

As time passed, the group became a lifeline for the members. Nobody missed a session. However, the sessions seemed all the same. They would talk about their life history, the hardships they had to face, both back in Turkey and in the UK, the difficulties of being an immigrant, their illnesses, their medications, their anxieties and so on. My interpretations about the fear of difference in the group fell on deaf ears. While they became comrades in arms, I felt increasingly isolated and concerned. Was I trying to do the impossible, running a group analytic group with a Turkish membership? Was I going against the grain? I was feeling stuck and tired. Despite trying, it had not been possible to bring in new members. The group was so enmeshed, including myself to some degree, that there was no room for anybody else.

The turning point

The turning point for the group was the week I had to cancel the group for the first time in the two and a half years it had been running due to a heavy flu. In the following session, there was mutiny in the group. They were all very angry with me, seemingly for phoning them to cancel the group. I had never seen them so animated. I thought that I must have done something very wrong but did not know what it could be. That was, until they spoke about the News about the two 6th-century monumental Buddha statues in Afghanistan, carved into the side of a cliff, being blown up by the terrorist group Taliban in 2001. There I was – the terrorist who blew up the Godly figure in the group, which they thought was built in stone, by revealing myself as a mere mortal, who had got ill. I was no longer omnipresent or omnipotent.

It took weeks for the group to recover. The members literally told me that I could never be the same again for them. The rage and the hatred towards me felt palpable. However, once the group settled, members began to talk about their differences and started to challenge each other. Also, I was able to bring in two new members. After the following break, there were no reports of hallucinations or the compilation of disasters that usually had occurred during the break.

In my 2003 paper, I had wondered about the long-term implications of this particular incident in the group (Sengun, 2003) and had thought 'maybe I was not going against the grain, but it took as long as two years to reach a certain developmental stage in the group as described in group analytic teaching'. It seems I was right. Not only did this culturally very different group slowly become like any other group, going through the usual group processes, but also it moved from strength to strength. The members learned to recognise feelings and how to express them, worked through trauma and abuse and gained self-esteem and confidence. In addition, they worked through the culture-specific group processes concerning authority, individuation and intimacy, as identified by Devan (2001).

The first member's leaving not only opened the way for the next member but also made me aware that they were all ready to leave but did not dare. As soon as I realised this, the possibility of ending the group occurred to me. It was a difficult decision to make, but I gave a year's notice to close down the group. The members worked through the ending without any major difficulties which confirmed their readiness to end therapy.

Some afterthoughts

Although this group became a success story at the end, it required a lot of patience and very hard work. Coming from the same culture, my own transferences and identifications were strong. The group stirred up a lot in me and I had to deal with my own dependency and separation issues. Running other clinical groups alongside with a diverse membership helped to balance my overall experience of groups. Weekly supervision was most necessary and being in therapy also helped greatly.

On the other hand, I learned so much from conducting this group. Not only did it enable me to work on myself, but also it helped me to develop a genuine cultural sensitivity. This sensitivity is not overly concerned with being politically correct, but it requires to have an ongoing awareness of the impact of culture on the individual and on the group. Developing such cultural sensitivity not only allowed me to openly question the impact of culture with other patients, including the ones who are from unfamiliar cultures, but also challenge what at times is presented as a cultural norm (Sengun, 1997). Simply accepting as a cultural norm what is presented, just because we do not understand the other's culture or because of the fear of not being politically correct, or in order to avoid conflict in the group, not only renders the group ineffective but also deprives its members of the opportunity to develop and to broaden their horizons. This is very different from imposing the conductor's culture or belief system or a 'Western' psychotherapy culture on the group. Is it not the case, that everyday group analysis questions and examines all social and cultural norms, regardless of where and with whom the group is held?

Acknowledgements

I would like to express my gratitude to Sue Einhorn for her invaluable supervision of the group and for her comments on this chapter. Also, many thanks to Jale Cilasun, a close friend and a colleague, for our ongoing discussion on culture, the social unconscious and everything else.

Chapter 8

Finding words for it – the birth of group analytic training in Rwanda

Justin Phipps

Introduction

Dawn breaks and the eerie sound of a woman's screams resound across the valley from my guesthouse in the Rwandan capital Kigali.

Checking out of my hotel, the tall young man on reception glances down at the register on the desk and as he does, I catch sight of the deep machete wound gouged in the top of his skull, inflicted two decades earlier.

Just two glimpses of the rawness and trauma that still lie beneath the surface today, more than twenty-five years after the genocide. With its nationwide broadband network and shiny new international conference centre, Kigali has many of the trappings of modernity. It is hard not to be impressed by the construction boom in the capital and recent levels of economic growth.

I first visited Rwanda in 1981, while working for an aid agency. I spent three weeks travelling round the rural areas of the country, which is only slightly larger than Wales. During the 1994 Genocide, I was far away in Britain, preoccupied with other work and bringing up a young family. But I remember my sense of intense shock on seeing BBC footage of the militias at roadblocks, routinely hacking people to death. In the course of one hundred days, between April and July 1994, hundreds of thousands of people were killed.

Almost twenty years later, in 2013, I returned to Rwanda having recently qualified as a Group Analyst. It was impossible not to be struck by the extraordinary changes in the country. The population had almost doubled to thirteen million and previously bare green hills were now covered with new houses and settlements. Under the Rwandan Patriotic Front and its leader, President Paul Kagame, Rwanda is attempting to build a new society that is prosperous, secure, clean and orderly. The refugee diaspora has returned to the urban centres and a new generation has grown up after the genocide.

Beginnings

In 2013, I began discussions with two local non-governmental organisations (NGOs) about the possibility of establishing a group analytic training

DOI: 10.4324/9781003310358-12

working with genocide survivors: the Survivors' Fund (SURF) and *Avega Agahozo* (Widows of the Genocide – 'Dry your tears'). It had struck me that, while many Rwandan NGOs were running counselling groups across the country, most of their staff were psychologists, who had received no specialist training in group psychotherapy.

On my return to Britain, I sounded out some colleagues about this idea and the following year went back to Rwanda as part of a team of group analysts to undertake a pilot week of training. Our staff team is made up of three people: Anne Morgan, who lives in South Africa, MJ Maher, who is of African origin, and me, white British: two women, one man; two white people (*Abazungu*), one black person; two Europeans, one African; each of us with different experiences of living or working in Africa.

Working in a team of three has felt creative, allowing for a range of differing perspectives, even if at times the triangular dynamic can also give rise to feelings of exclusion or rivalry. Seeing how differently people react to the three of us, we have been able to think about race and gender. Between visits, we have had regular supervision with Elisabeth Rohr, a senior German group analyst, where we can explore the impact of the work on us personally.

Rwanda

Rwanda – 'The land of a thousand hills' – is a small, densely populated country in the Great Lakes region of East and Central Africa. It is a highly organised society, where the population can be easily mobilised. Before – and during – the colonial period, the country was a monarchy, with a divine king, the Tutsi *Mwami*, presiding over a court and an array of military, land and cattle chiefs. It was a hierarchical, pyramidal system, with eighteen patrilineal clans distributed across the country.

In 'The Premise of Inequality in Ruanda', Jacques Maquet describes how young warriors (the *Intore*) were selected to be socialised in the values of the court and were given practical training in self-mastery (*Itonde*). Everyone aspired to be dignified, reserved and polite. It was shameful to lose one's temper or manifest strong emotions (Maquet, 1961, p. 118). A system of patron-client relations operated, governing access to land and cattle. Under *Ubuhake*, clients could normally use their patrons' cows and benefit from usufruct and grazing rights in return for the performance of services. There was an element of reciprocity to this, which contrasted strongly with the *Uburetwa* system of forced labour.

At the end of the 19th century, Rwanda became part of German East Africa, then after the First World War, came under Belgian administration, first under a League of Nations mandate, and from 1920, as part of a UN trust territory Ruanda-Urundi. In 1961, Rwanda became a Republic and finally achieved independence from Belgium in July 1962.

During the colonial period ethnic divisions were fostered and accentuated, with the introduction of identity cards, and after independence power passed to Hutu regimes under Grégoire Kayibanda (1961–1973) and Juvénal Habyarimana (1973–1994). The period leading up to the Genocide was marked by a move towards a multi-party political system and an economic crisis linked to a collapse in the price of coffee. This combined with the manipulation of a sense of historic grievance by the political elite and the emergence of an explicitly racist ideology directed against the Tutsi minority. During the genocide, terror and coercion were used to eliminate all opposition and the general population was initiated into violence, leading to the erosion of any taboos against cruelty and sadism.

Language and the problems of translation

Unlike many African countries, Rwanda has a single local language, Kinyarwanda, although most people also speak some English, French or Kiswahili. Under Belgian colonial rule, the official language was French. More recently, English has been adopted, influenced by the number of returning refugees, who grew up in exile in Anglophone countries such as Uganda, as well as by Rwanda's decision to join the East African Community.

The training courses have been run in the participants' mother tongue, using three local interpreters. Their standard of interpreting is high. Holding regular meetings has been important, enabling us to gain insights into Rwandan society. There have also been times when the interpreters have been profoundly affected by some of the traumatic material in the small groups, for example, when this had echoes of their own personal experience of the genocide. Working with interpreters, I have found that my understanding of the details of what is said often has to be sacrificed in the interests of letting the group conversation flow naturally in the students' mother tongue. A salutary reminder of how much we always miss as conductors.

'For which purpose?'

As a staff team we have been conscious of how, in Africa, foreigners are seen through the twin lenses of race and colonialism. *Abazungu* (white people) come and go, invariably promising and failing to deliver. Having an African member of the team has made a huge difference through helping us to think more deeply about local beliefs, as well as revisiting attitudes towards *Abazungu*.

In his article 'Socio-Cultural Influence on Group Therapy Leadership Style', Mohammed Taha compares the "more directive, prescriptive and active leadership style" he is familiar with in Egypt, with "the less directive, more descriptive and passive style that was developed in the UK" (Taha et al., 2008). He questions how far the latter is appropriate in his own country.

We were uncertain whether this might also be the case in Rwanda, where there are clear expectations of authority, dating back to the hierarchical patron-client relations of the pre-colonial court. How far should we stay faithful to our training and how far would we need to adapt to the local context?

The initial reaction to our group analytic way of working was one of confusion. There were two aspects to this. First, the lack of an explicit agenda. To many course participants, a free-floating conversation seemed aimless and lacking in direction. The students were used to a formal, didactic style of teaching and were disoriented by a more experiential form of learning. In the words of one participant: "For which purpose?"

Second, there was also mystification at the apparent absence of strong leadership in a society used to deferring to authority. This made me think again about Foulkes' comment about the group being "weaned from the infantile need for authoritative guidance" (Foulkes, 1964, p. 61) and "dependence upon authority [being] replaced by reliance on the strength of the group itself" (Foulkes, 1964, p. 63).

Trauma

Ukize inkuba árayigànìra – To escape thunder is to speak about it (Danger can only be talked about once it is over) (Crépeau and Bizimana, 1979, p. 446).

The majority of our students were born before the 1994 Genocide, but many were still young children or teenagers at the time. It is hard to conceive what they endured or the indescribable horrors they witnessed. It is in the nature of trauma that the part of the self that is emotionally overwhelmed becomes split off. This enables another part to function and survive.

In her unpublished paper 'Trauma and Refugees', Farideh Dizadji (2016) refers to the work of the Hungarian psychoanalyst Sandor Ferenczi, who saw fragmentation as a useful defence in surviving trauma. She writes:

> The task is to overcome the fragmentation, to overcome trauma. However it is nearly impossible to deal with trauma in such a linear manner, because 'within' the traumatic experience, there are only pains, no words, and no capacity for thinking reflectively. 'Outside' of the trauma, thinking, works and words exist, but without being totally connected to the traumatic experiences.
>
> (Dizadji, 2016, p. 10)

She goes on to say that in working with traumatised people, it's essential to take account of the 'double-reality' they experience:

> On one side there is a person who can talk about, think about, and even tell us about what happened to them. On the other side, we have a

person lost in the experience of death and terror, for whom there are no words to explain their experience.

(Dizadji, 2016, p. 10)

During the training in Rwanda, we have been struck by how frequently students displayed somatic symptoms. We also noticed, when visiting groups run by local NGOs, that they often incorporate music, dancing and prayer into sessions, and this appears to alleviate some of the traumatic symptoms. Following our pilot visit, we decided to include body relaxation techniques in the course program. We drew on materials originally developed by the NHS, but then encouraged the students to improvise their own exercises, games and drama.

In Western Europe, psychodynamic therapy is usually viewed as 'talking therapy'. There is, for example, a taboo on touching. But in Rwanda, as in many other parts of Africa, a simple mind-body distinction makes little sense, as people's conception of the world tends to be more integrated and holistic. The mind is inseparable from the body, just as the individual is inseparable from the group and society, to which they belong. A good illustration of this is the Southern African concept of *Ubuntu* – it is other people who make us who we are. So it has been crucial for us constantly to question our assumptions and try to look at things afresh.

Rwandan NGOs

Given the shortage of local opportunities for therapy, many of our students have thrown themselves into work with NGOs. Rwandan NGOs tend to fall into two broad categories, those that work with groups exclusively composed of survivors and those who are involved in reconciliation work with mixed groups of perpetrators and survivors.

One of the remarkable features about Rwanda is the way, in which perpetrators and survivors still live side by side, in close proximity to each other. Attending local groups where both participate can be an extraordinary experience. It set me thinking about the title of Philip Gourevitch's forthcoming book about survivors and perpetrators *You hide that you hate me, I hide that I know* (Gourevitch, to be published 2023).

Evolution of the training

The first Rwandan Group Analytic Foundation Course ran from June 2016 to November 2017. A second course, together with a concurrent new Intermediate Course, began in 2019 and these two courses are still in progress. The training has been held at the AVEGA conference centre in Rwamagana, in the East of the country, as a week-long residential course that takes place twice yearly over a period of two years. At any one time, we have about thirty students, two-thirds of whom are women. Together with our staff team and the three interpreters, this makes a total of thirty-six people.

After the initial shock of adapting to a new way of working, we have found our students to be very appreciative of the space offered by the small groups. Most of them had rarely discussed their genocide experience openly with others, and few, if any, have had the opportunity of personal therapy. Over time, there has been a shift in the small groups from a discussion of the students' work to a disclosure of more personal experiences.

In Rwanda, people are accustomed to telling their stories in the form of formal genocide testimonies and there can be an expectation that this is what outsiders want to hear. This tendency, combined with a social norm of hearing people out or letting them have their say, has at times proved a difficult combination. To have to cut people off in mid-flow may seem disrespectful, but a group analytic conversation or discussion does not sit easily with lengthy monologues. As the courses have evolved, our small groups have begun to talk about a wider range of subjects, such as rites of passage, like births, weddings and funerals, or burglaries, eating disorders and so on.

The large group in the training

By contrast, our students remain puzzled by the large group. Again, this is partly due to the apparent lack of any agenda and the perceived failure of staff to lead the discussion.

The large group sessions have been very lively, with relatively little silence. They are often accompanied by what I have come to think of as 'the buzz' – an audible 'hum' as people react to what is discussed and turn to their neighbours and comment. The power of large groups was shown, when, on the final day of our pilot visit, one of the students was re-traumatised and this, in turn, triggered a traumatic reaction in others present, although the way in which the students collectively handled the situation was impressive. Following this experience, we decided to move the final large group session to the penultimate day of the course.

We have found that in the large group, issues of leadership and status come to the fore, and male students tend to become more vocal. There is also a prevalent anxiety about conflict erupting, which could leave individuals feeling isolated, exposed or scapegoated. The church plays an important role in Rwanda and the complex interplay between Christianity and other local spiritual beliefs has also been apparent. Subjects like witchcraft can be divisive, polarising opinion, while dreams, with their predictive power, are capable of inspiring real terror.

Indirect communication and the use of proverbs (Imigani)

"'A message is given to many, but those who are meant to understand, understand'. There's always a subtext in Rwanda. You don't have to resort to brutal language. People understand" (Alison DesForges, cited in the *New York Times* (McNeil, 2002, 17th March)).

As the training has evolved, we have become aware as a staff team how easy it is for us to fail to pick up on the subtext in the groups, to miss anger, or misinterpret laughter. The Rwandan psychologist Déogratias Bagilishya has emphasised the role of proverbs and non-verbal gestures in mourning and coming to terms with loss:

> In Rwandan tradition the proverb is a mode of communication often used to express what a person has seen, heard and experienced at the level of emotions, feelings and states of mind, as well as to indicate to someone that they have been understood.
>
> (Bagilishya, 2000, p. 342)

> The Kinyarwanda word *Imigani* ... expresses the notion of a conversation or dialogue, attempting to elicit 'a mode of expression used to recognise, confirm and participate in what the other is living on an emotional level'.
>
> (Bagilishya, cited in Uwihoreye and Pells, 2020)

In a society where communication is often indirect, proverbs leave scope for ambiguity and shades of meaning (Pells et al., 2021). During the training, we have noticed how frequently they are used in what remains a predominantly oral culture. It has also occurred to us that proverbs are almost impossible to translate and so may also sometimes offer a convenient way of excluding foreigners. By their nature, proverbs are both elusive and paradoxical. But they also represent two-way communication, connecting the speaker with the audience by invoking a shared reference point. There are many Rwandan proverbs that relate to communication and secrecy. Some suggest that openness is desirable:

> *Utaganiriye na se ntamenya icyosekuru yasize avuze.* If you don't talk with your father, you cannot know what your grandfather said before dying.
>
> (Uwihoreye and Pells, 2020)

And that conversation can lead to greater openness:

> *Ukuri gushirira mu biganiro.* The truth always emerges through conversation.
>
> (Truth will out)

But speaking out can also sometimes have terrible consequences.

> *Akarenze impinga karushya ihamagara.* What reaches the brow of the hill cannot be recalled.
>
> (Crépeau and Bizimana, 1979, p. 81)

It therefore makes sense to bottle things up inside. *Uhishe munda imbwa ntimwiba.* Dogs can't steal what you hide inside. (If you reveal something, there is a risk of everyone knowing, whereas no one can know what is concealed within).

Secrecy (*Ibanga*) is prized in Rwanda and seen as valuable in itself. In the past, a form of blood brotherhood existed, known as *Igihango* (trust). This was a secret pact of friendship, which helped forge social bonds between families. Such secrets, sealed with blood, were never to be revealed. But over time secrets can become burdensome and there is a danger of their being revealed to others. A Rwandan saying describes someone who, having guarded a secret for a very long time, stores it in a hole in the ground, for safekeeping. But the echo reverberates, and others get to hear of it (*Gucukura akobo umuntu aka kongorera ibanga*).

At first sight, group analysis may appear diametrically opposed to Rwandan culture, but I believe it is simplistic to see it in those terms. Group analysis provides a flexible way of working, which takes account of the social and political context, while Rwandan culture is more fluid and changing than sometimes portrayed. Within group analysis, it is generally seen as axiomatic that increased openness is a desirable goal. Foulkes saw mental health problems as closely linked to blocked communication and inseparable from the fundamentally social nature of human beings. For him articulating the unconscious at a conscious level was a prime objective. In *Therapeutic Group Analysis* (Foulkes, 1964), he defines translation as "the equivalent of making conscious of the repressed unconscious in psycho-analysis" (Foulkes, 1964, p. 111).

In our Rwanda training, it seems that openness and secrecy go hand in hand, the verbal with the non-verbal, the mind and the body together.

Conclusion

> *Agahinda kinkono kamenywa n'uwayiharuye.* The sorrow of a cooking pot is understood by the person, who has scraped its bottom. (One can only help others by genuinely listening to their suffering).
>
> (Bagilishya, 2000, p. 341)

Six years after embarking on the Rwandan training, we need to be cautious about reaching any definitive conclusions. The residential setting and the professional links between students have helped to establish a sense of trust and togetherness. We have also noticed a high level of mutual support at times of illness or family crisis, and this has helped alleviate our initial concern about how they would manage in the relatively long gaps between our visits.

Our students are highly motivated and show enthusiasm and commitment. They seem to have a capacity to think symbolically in a way not often seen when conducting groups in Britain. It is interesting to speculate on the reasons for this and whether it might, in some way, be linked to a culture of indirect communication – although that is often said to be a feature of British society too.

As outsiders, we need to be clear about the limits to our ability to read emotions or to understand the sub-text of what is being said. We are after all working in another language, using interpreters, and Rwanda has an extremely complex political history.

Writing this paper, it has often been difficult to find words to describe our experience adequately. This mirrors the experience of the students, who, after enduring the trauma of living through the genocide, still find it difficult to articulate their experience. Traumatic wounds take many years to heal, since it means reintegrating the part that is emotionally overwhelmed with the part that continues to survive and function.

Group analysis is adaptable and can be applied in many different social contexts; however, our experience in Rwanda suggests that it may be important to think again about the assumption that open communication is a straightforward or unambiguous objective. I have tried to show how in a culture where people are constrained from expressing themselves openly, secrets form an important element in social relations and proverbs and non-verbal communication can play a significant role when people tend to express themselves indirectly.

Acknowledgements

I would like to thank all our students, past and present, whose courage and insight have helped me to understand more about Rwanda. Thanks also to our interpreters and to our friends at the Survivors' Fund, AVEGA and all the other Rwandan NGOs, who have so generously given of their time and hospitality.

Finally, I want to thank my colleagues Anne Morgan and MJ Maher for their friendship, wisdom and ideas. From the outset, we have shared so much in our work together, but the views expressed in this chapter are my own.

Chapter 9

The dynamics of the social unconscious at work in the therapy group

Sylvia Hutchinson

Introduction

Anniversaries mark a point in time, usually a point of significant change, the birth of something new, the death of something old. Much has changed for the Warsaw Institute, not least due to the change of Poland's status in joining the European Union. It seemed appropriate to commemorate this anniversary with some reflections on change in the development of group analysis. Foulkes (1948, 1964, 1975) in his development of group analysis combined the language of psychoanalysis with that of social psychology, sociology, gestalt, systems and communications theory. Psychoanalytic language, with its extensive vocabulary and syntax, has been the dominant language system in group analysis. In the past twenty years or so, the language of group analysis has significantly increased its references to the social and the social unconscious – it has in fact enlarged its vocabulary of the social. This changing landscape sometimes provokes conflict between those who fear the corruption or atrophy of our psychoanalytic muscle and those who challenge its orthodoxy.

In the 1980s and 1990s, the work of the European Association of Trans-cultural Group Analysis (EATGA) (Brown, 2001), which organised intercultural groups to explore the dynamics of socio-cultural, ethnic, language and other differences, heightened our awareness of variation and difference and enhanced our understanding of such effects. In recent years, articles have appeared on social class (Blackwell, 2002; Storck, 2002), gender (Burman, 2002) and immigration (Bledin, 2003; Rohr, 2002; Sengun, 2001), emphasising the importance of the social context and its defining influence, in both its current and historical sense. But the question of how we work with the social unconscious in ordinary clinical situations remains elusive. This is the question I wish to address in this chapter.

In order to introduce the notion of the social unconscious, I would like to briefly recount one of my most memorable group experiences.

At the age of about fifteen, in the early part of my adolescence in Cape Town, South Africa, I was part of a small group, a breakaway youth movement group. The leader of this group, a lawyer who was keen to educate us,

DOI: 10.4324/9781003310358-13

occasionally brought his political friends to talk to us. There were about eight of us in the group and on one occasion, a black lawyer came and led a seminar on African history. Although I now remember little of the content of the seminar, I have a vivid memory of what I experienced as a transform-ative exchange. During the seminar, whilst discussing something or other, I referred to the 'garden boy'. Tulani, the black lawyer, very gently asked me why I referred to a fully grown man as a 'boy'? Instantaneously, I was aware that I would never dream of referring to a white man working in the garden as a 'garden boy'. I would instead refer to him as a gardener. Referring to blacks as boys or girls was common parlance amongst whites in South Af-rica. Despite regarding myself at that time as relatively self-aware, as well as aware of the deep injustice and cruelty of the apartheid regime and the des-perate clinging to power of the whites in South Africa, I was shocked to find myself part of that process, the process of infantilising and disempowering blacks – something that was quite outside my conscious awareness. This was for me a very personal experience of the social unconscious made conscious through an analysis of how it was embedded in language.

Group analysis – working with the social unconscious

The group analytic method, the creation and maintenance of a group ana-lytic situation and setting, and the maintenance of a 'group analytic attitude' by the conductor, provides an enduring and constant frame, unchanged by changing contexts. It is an analytic method which promotes access to uncon-scious dynamics. As group conductors, we 'seed and grow' a dynamic ma-trix and then it can be viewed from different observation points but always locating meaning in context, the dynamic context, the current social context and the historical context. But how do we view the social unconscious?

I have heard from group analysts, especially from immigrants in groups composed of those from the local home culture, that they have not ad-dressed or worked with their distinctive socio-cultural or political back-ground, when they were in their group analytic therapy. I include myself in this group, and I am amazed that this somehow never arose as an issue in any significant way.

This leaves me with a question: Does the group analytic method invar-iably provide access not only to the personal, repressed unconscious, but also to the internalised contemporary and historical socio-cultural forces shaping our development, the social unconscious? Or does it reduce or even obscure such access? Is access obscured not just for immigrants, but in a more general sense? If the absence of dialogue about socio-cultural back-ground is not an artefact of our method, could it be the case that in having an 'isolate', that is, an immigrant in the group, that the dominant majority culture calls for adaptation and acculturation? Foulkes cautioned against 'singular' group members, because the group may colonise the isolate, who may very well wish to be colonised and acculturated. Although members of a therapy group are of equal status, power differences between individuals and between subgroups are bound to emerge.

The social unconscious – power relations and differentials

My interest in the relationship between the psyche and the social and the use and abuse of power goes back a long way. After emigrating from South Africa to the UK in 1969, my first proper job was a one-year junior research fellowship at Sussex University in what was then called 'The Research Centre for Collective Psychopathology'. This research centre was set up to investigate how persecutions and exterminations came about, how the impulse to persecute and exterminate is generated and how it spreads. I participated in a field study on race relations which attempted to show how racial groups come to use and misuse each other. Now more than thirty years on, I find myself still preoccupied with the relationship between the psyche and the social world.

The publication of 'The Psyche and the Social World' (Brown and Zinkin, 1993) represented one of the first attempts to critically examine group analytic theory and practice. Since then, alongside Nitsun's (1996) anti-group challenge to Foulkes' possible blind spots, there have been in recent years a number of authors such as Farhad Dalal (1998), Earl Hopper (2003a) and Ralph Stacey (2001), who have presented challenges to the theoretical base and the underlying paradigms of group analysis, all paying particular attention to the notion of the social unconscious. I wonder if it is noteworthy that all these authors, like Foulkes, are immigrants practicing in a host country that is not their country of origin.

Hopper and Dalal approach the social unconscious from different angles. Dalal assumes the position of a critical theorist attempting to elaborate and extend what he has called 'radical' Foulksian theory. Hopper speaks as clinician and theorist emphasising the importance and relative neglect of the social unconscious in the analytic field and proposes a model for how to work with it in a clinical context. Stacey's view, which I cannot elaborate on here, has much in common with Dalal, but does not see the need for recourse to a notion of the social unconscious, as he eschews any idea of a determining or causal force whether arising from the individual or the social. Although a number of other authors (Brown, 2001; Fromm, 1999) have contributed to ideas on the social unconscious, I will focus on the work of Dalal and Hopper for the present purpose.

Dalal's view of the social unconscious

Dalal (1998) challenges the orthodoxy of reducing the social to the individual. He makes a distinction between the notion that an individual is affected by their socio-cultural system and the notion that the unconscious is as such structured by the social. Through careful text analysis of Foulkes' writings, he identifies two versions of Foulkes' notion of the social unconscious. Firstly orthodox Foulkes, who retains the notion of the individual, Freudian unconscious as distinct from the social unconscious, the social made unconscious. Secondly radical Foulkes, where all inner processes and structures are permeated by group or social forces, that is, the social permeates the deepest level of the psyche including the 'id'.

By developing 'radical' Foulkes in connection with the ideas of Norbert Elias, Dalal (1998) builds a case for a recursive model, in which individuals simultaneously and reciprocally construct and are constructed by the social. Here individual and social, nature and nurture, conscious and unconscious, are embedded in each other and cannot be reduced one to the other. Following Elias, he identifies power relations and power differentials as the prime factor shaping the particular manifestations of the social unconscious. Dalal then teases out some implications of his argument for clinical method. Most significant amongst these, in my view, is the need to take greater account of power differentials influencing the therapeutic relationship, as reflected in the psyches of its participants. His version, which I am closest to, defines the unconscious as permeated by the social – the social unconscious being embedded in and manifesting itself through language, thought processes and communication networks.

Hopper's view of the social unconscious

Hopper defines the social unconscious differently as follows:

> The concept of the social unconscious refers to the existence and constraints of social, cultural and communication arrangements of which people are unaware.
>
> (Hopper, 2003, p. 127)

While this may seem quite consistent with Dalal's version and his elaboration of a recursive model, Dalal identifies now and again a tendency in Hopper's writing to reduce the social to the individual.

Hopper takes the concept into the clinical field by suggesting that no transference interpretation is complete without considering the defining effects of social-historical facts and forces.

> An analyst who is unaware of the effect of social facts and social forces will not be sensitive to the unconscious recreation of them within the therapeutic situation. He will not be able to provide a space for patients to imagine how their identities have been formed at particular historical and political junctures, and how this continues to affect them throughout their lives.
>
> (Hopper, 2003, p. 126)

Hopper thus provides a frame of reference for clinical work. In particular, for the completion of work with the transference by extending Malan's (1979) 'therapeutic triangle' by linking the 'here and now' of the therapeutic relationship to the 'here and then' of past early significant relationships, and to the 'there and now' of current significant relationships. He extends this therapeutic triangle to a 'therapeutic square' by including working with the 'there and then', referring to the patient's early experience of social facts and forces in the past, usually mediated through the family and other early primary groups. Hopper suggests that working with the 'there and then' and the 'now and there', that is, with current social or interpersonal networks of relationships, will provide the necessary access to the social unconscious.

Rouchy (1995), a founder member of the European Association of Transcultural Group Analysis, distinguishes between the 'natural' group of primary belonging, that is the family and significant others connected to the family, and 'instituted' groups of secondary belonging, which are instituted groups in which people are brought together, like school groups, work groups, professional groups and so on. According to him, cultural internalisation is completed by these secondary belonging groups, which have the function of socialisation and the internalisation of norms and values. But there is a danger if these groups do not take on this function or pervert it

> as in totalitarian regimes, [where] groups of secondary belonging can become threatening and persecuting, provoking identity conflicts and a fragmentation of identity. Continuity or discontinuity between groups of primary and secondary belonging are thus one of the determining factors in the structuralisation of identity and its misadventures.
>
> (Rouchy, 1995, p. 137)

The psychoanalytic tradition has tended to constrain the understanding of the transference to the primary belonging groups, the family. A fuller understanding of transference would need to take the possible conflicts and discontinuities in the experience of primary and secondary belonging groups and their effects on identity formation into account. The conductor and members of a therapy group may act as transference triggers for parental and other family members, but they may also represent social roles that trigger transference reactions. Roles that signify location and status in the social and power hierarchy, such as the employer, the boss, the teacher, the politician, the professional, the worker, the student, the housewife. Transference reactions may also represent or stand for particular groups and/or ideologies, like the conservatives, the working classes, the feminists, the blacks, the radicals and so on. Exclusive attention to transferences from the primary family group may obscure a more comprehensive understanding of the dynamics of individuals in relationship.

Working with the social unconscious in therapy groups

Hopper's formulation directs us to how we might work with the social unconscious, but it does not give any indicators as to 'when' such work is necessary. The group-analytic method is non-directive. The conductor follows the group and only intervenes when there are blockages in communication and a need to help translate communications into more easily shareable forms. I believe Hopper's formulation in directing us to the 'there and then' allows the conductor too much room to set the agenda. I would like to bring an example from one of my therapy groups to take these ideas on how and when we might access the social unconscious forward. In the following clinical illustrations, names have been changed and personal identifying information eliminated.

Clinical example (1)

In a slow-open once-weekly group with seven members, themes of manipulative and exploitative relationships recurred over an extended period. At the time, analytic reflections in the group were primarily confined to transference analysis relating to family dynamics and the analysis of projective systems. A retrospective look at the dynamics of this group now suggests an incomplete analysis. This group had an interesting and diverse mix of cultures, including Italian, Greek-Cypriot, German, English and Irish.

Peter, a responsive and provocative presence in the group, brings his intense need and hunger for soothing. He has just looked after his daughter who stays with him for alternate weekends. Peter is English and from a middle-class background. He came into therapy to work on his difficulties in intimate relationships with women. He described a highly conflictual relationship with his mother who set him up as capable of unlimited achievements, yet constantly accused him of selfish and manipulative behaviour, particularly when failing to attend to her needs.

Maria (second generation Greek-Cypriot) responds to Peter's request for soothing and comfort by questioning his sense of entitlement and by challenging his demands, which she views as draining the group just as he feels drained. Maria, attractive, articulate and competent, came into group to work on her anxieties about intimate sexual relationships. She felt controlled and dominated by her mother, who had discouraged close contact with peers for fear of their contaminating influence. Maria was ashamed of her body and her lack of intimate sexual experience and tended to defend against feared rejection by critical attack.

Peter pleads with the group for a shared experience of need and finds solace in Sally, whom he identifies as the one most like him, who is able to own and express her needs. Sally (English) was regarded by her siblings as spoilt but experienced herself as deprived of warmth and nurturance.

In the weeks that follow, Maria shows increasing sensitivity to any inattention, sharpness or slight from Peter, culminating in an angry outburst following Peter's declaration that he is attracted to and likes Sally, who he feels supports him. Sally responds positively expressing appreciation of his presence in and contribution to the group, whilst Maria condemns this behaviour as unacceptable and divisive. The group-as-a-whole explores feelings associated with pairing and rivalry, jealousy and exclusion in terms of both sibling and oedipal constellations, both in the group, in relation to me, and in current and past family relationships.

Over the weeks that follow, Maria repeatedly brings into the group her conviction that in Peter's presence, she cannot effectively use the group. She feels dismissed and disregarded by him and only feels safe in the group in his very occasional absence. With mounting rage, she attributes to him all that is selfish and manipulative and sees him as feeding his sexualised need for intimacy by using others as objects, and that her only defence is to withhold those aspects of herself that she most needs to disclose in order to use the group therapeutically. Peter is stunned, at first takes it on the chin, valuing her 'honesty' in bringing what she really feels, and sharing his concern that what she has expressed is what he most fears about himself. He also makes some attempts to separate himself from her projections onto him.

The group divides in its emotional alliances, with Sally in support of Peter, and Sian (from an Irish, catholic, working-class background) strongly supporting Maria. Other members keep out of the conflict, some visibly frightened by it.

In a session where Maria brings her feelings about Peter's inhibitory effect on her and Peter identifies her as communicating in a way uncannily close to his mother's treatment of him – using the same words 'selfish and manipulative', as the group draws to a close, Peter becomes tearful and talks about how vulnerable he feels and how painful he is finding this experience. He asks Maria to be gentle with him, to which she responds that she can't pretend or control the way she feels. At the end, he turns to Sally and says that it would really help him if she gave him a hug. She declines graciously.

The following session Maria begins with apologies to Sally by citing this event as evidence of Peter's manipulative control. No holds barred, she says her worst, telling Peter that she sees him as abusive and perverse. Peter defends himself, disclaiming the character that Maria describes him as, but again owning his fear of these aspects in himself. The group protects Peter by focusing on Maria, providing an alternative perspective on Peter and attempting to correct her transference distortions. As the heat reduces, Maria offers Peter her recognition that her view may not reflect who he actually is. After some delay, Peter responds by attempting to secure and control what she has just offered, asking for more of it and for its confirmation. In this, he repeats his defensive attempts to control his mother's response to him. The full cycle of this dynamic interplay is now articulated in the group: Maria in her mother's attacking and controlling voice defends against injury to her fragile self, whilst Peter in his attempts to control his self-objects recreates his relationship with his controlling mother.

Around this time, a new member, Janet (English, middle class background), joins the group. Over the coming months, Maria withdraws her feelings of hate from Peter and transfers them to Janet, again with Sian as her ally and in strong support. She repeats the cycle of verbal attack, accusing Janet of manipulation and exploitation and of inhibiting her from using the group.

Peter, and a few weeks later Maria, leave the group, Peter with a good and well worked-through ending – and Maria with a strong attack on me in her last group (with Janet absent) for having been blinded and duped by 'mad' Janet and for being at the mercy of her sinister manipulations. The group challenges Maria, pointing to her capacity for destructive attack – she responds with a clear statement that she embraces being able to fight and wouldn't want to lose her capacity to use words as weapons.

Discussion of example (1)

Maria claimed to have gained some therapeutic benefit from the group, though in my view, this was relatively limited. Instead of reaching for explanations in terms of her capacity to use dynamic therapy, as I did at the time, I wonder now whether a closer look at the social unconscious and internalised power relations may have offered possibilities to shift the exploitative dynamic that Maria was caught up in.

Subgroup formation

An analysis of relatively enduring subgroup formations throws up the following interesting configurations. Maria (second generation Greek-Cypriot) and Sian (second generation Irish) constituted the subgroup that persistently attacked, with accusations of sinister exploitation and manipulation, the English subgroup, first Peter and then Janet (both of relatively high social status) with Sally in alliance. Maria and Sian (with their roots in Cyprus and Ireland) share in their socio-political background a history of a colonial relationship with England, in which England had the power to occupy or withdraw, provide or exploit. The two remaining group members, both born in the years following World War II, were immigrants from Germany and Italy, countries that had been at war with England, embattled and ultimately defeated. Both these men expressed their anxiety at the continuing conflict and attack in the group and on the whole attempted to keep out and not take sides in the conflict, though there seemed to be an implicit vicarious satisfaction in witnessing the attacks. It is interesting to speculate as to whether a transference analysis that extended back to the relevant formative socio-political contexts and power configurations may have facilitated some further transformation of the dynamics of the group and the individuals in it.

I myself, representing the subgroup 'Conductor', was accused by Maria in her final session of being the 'blind witness' to exploitation and sinister manipulations, a particularly potent attack in terms of my own background having grown up as a privileged white South African, bearing witness to terrible oppression enacted in my name. Was I in feeling protective of those repeatedly attacked in the group, also protecting myself from the guilt and shame of power abuse?

Working with the social unconscious in therapy groups

The analysis of the above example suggests that subgroup formation and the lines that demarcate them may cue us into the social unconscious. Enduring subgroup formations indicate a blockage in communication, as they undermine free floating discussion, and may signal the need for analysis of the underlying social facts and forces and their particular power-relational configurations. Any demarcation of difference contains a potential power differential. Potential subgroup formations can take an infinite number of forms, based on identification of behaviour, affect states, attitudes, values and so on. Subgroups that form along lines of gender, sexuality, class, colour, ethnicity, language, culture, nationality or other social factors, are implicitly or explicitly concerned with power relations. In the above example, the subgroup Maria and Sian had social histories of being colonised, of migration and of having to adapt to the culture of an imperialist power. For Maria, the 'instituted groups of secondary belonging', that is school, university and work groups were presented to her in the family as potentially corrupting and exploitative and were then experienced as such by her. The subgroup representing the English, with their relatively high status and power in the social hierarchy, provided a ready target for the transference of such expectations. If subgroups had been identified at the time, facilitating a discussion in this way of where one was located in the power hierarchy and how that may have affected identity formation, I wonder now whether this may have allowed for an amelioration of the exploitative dynamic that shaped Maria's ongoing relationships. I would like briefly to look at one final example from a different group.

Clinical example (2)

In a group with six members, all raised in England but with varied religious and cultural backgrounds, the majority subgroup was from very deprived working-class backgrounds. Tanya was raised by a single mother who was

considered unsuitable to parent adolescent children, resulting in Tanya going into care when she reached puberty. Her mother was alienated from her
community and appeared to have no alternative 'belonging groups'. Tanya's
experience of her mother as inadequate, chaotic and needy left her with a
residue of deep mistrust and fear of intimacy which expressed itself as a
fear of the neediness and demands of others. The institution of the National
Health Service, which Tanya had made extensive use of, provided an alternative care-taking and maternal function, and educational institutions
provided the main channel for her to develop her resources and empower
herself. She had managed through her driving ambition to educate herself
and acquire knowledge and qualifications, to work and to support herself
working with the learning disabled. She was strongly aligned with the workers, anti-establishment and highly politicised. She had chronic difficulties in
all her work relationships, frequently alienating her colleagues. Apart from
one lengthy past relationship, in which she was cared for and supported, she
has avoided any intimate attachments.

Tanya soon established herself as the social historian and political commentator in the group. She compulsively responded to any contributions
that hinted at prejudice or stereotyping and in particular the use and abuse
of power by those in authority roles, usually with a lecture on class conflict or with a commentary on past or present political situations. Her un-
empathic responses often ruptured the ongoing emotional connections in
the group. The group, somewhat intimidated by Tanya, nevertheless resisted
the pressure towards 'political correctness'. On occasions, I would point out
how Tanya used her ideological stance defensively to avoid intimacy and
would link it to her anxieties about attaching to the group and her early
experience of failed dependency. The group would affirm her in her chosen
political role and encourage her political ambitions whilst resisting her misuse of this in the context of the group and her attempts to control the group.
But this did not shift the pattern.

After some months and mounting frustration, a group member whom
Tanya had been most closely aligned with as a fellow member of the working classes, got angry with her over assumptions Tanya had made about
her feminist ideology. Other members joined in and Tanya, upset and angry, and accusing the whole group of being a bunch of white, middle-class
oppressors, stormed out of the group five minutes before the end. On her
return, the following week the group took up issues of class, some challenging Tanya's stereotypes and two members talking in depth about their
own experience of growing up on the margins of society, without even a
solid working-class culture to belong to. Others in the group defended their
middle-class status, denying any intentional misuse of power but acknowledging the potential for it. This was a transformative time for Tanya and the
group. It allowed the group to explore in depth their positioning and their
mobility in the class and power structure and how this had affected them.

It also encouraged Tanya to move out of her rigid and defended position and into a dialogue with others. In the following weeks, she talked about improvements in her relationships at work and about her feeling that she was benefitting from being in the group.

For Tanya, 'instituted groups of secondary belonging', the care home and the educational and health institutions, were primary sources of socialisation and survival. She constructed her world according to those who had power and influence and those who didn't. Through an enactment of class warfare in the group and the mirroring of some aspects of her experience by two other members, her either/or views of the group and the social world were modified, and she could take further steps towards attaching to the group and feeling part of it. This is an example of how, without any specific direction from the conductor, the group accessed their 'there and then' experiences of the social worlds that had in the past shaped their development.

Conclusion

It seems to me that in groups with therapeutic aims, there is no need to actively direct attention to the social unconscious. Foulkes stipulates that the conductor should not lead the group but should be responsive to the group and its servant, rather than its master and should be mindful of the enormous power invested in him and not misuse it.

The transference patterns of communication will carry within them the unconscious socio-cultural and communicational arrangements and constraints – arrangements that organise our thinking and language – and these will manifest in the communications and enactments in the group. The 'here and now' communications and enactments in the group will, for the most part, remain unconscious. When they become configured into fixed or persistent patterns, the work of analysing and translating from one context to another is called for. Exclusive attention to the transference of early family relationships without contextualising the family in its past social milieu may obscure or even prevent access to the social unconscious. This reduces possibilities for shared understanding. Considering the transferences in a more general sense allows for the language of the social to be more fully incorporated. An increased awareness of the significance of cultural and socio-political forces in identity formation should enable group analysts to be more sensitive to their manifestation in the group. If the therapeutic experience in training does not encompasses such awareness, other consciousness-raising possibilities are essential. The large group in training may provide a good structure for such a purpose.

A number of contemporary psychoanalytic approaches, for instance, intersubjectivity or relational approaches, attachment theory and self-psychology, have adopted relational paradigms that have much in common with the group analytic approach. Some have also moved towards taking account of the social. I believe that group analysis has led the way in this respect – and is leading the way in the attempt to bring the social into clinical practice. Nevertheless, we still have some way to go in establishing an approach that fully takes account of the effects and the permeating power of the social.

Chapter 10

Who helps whom? – a group analytic approach to working with mothers and babies in an NHS perinatal mental health service

Sheila Ritchie

> As soon as they see the words 'mental health' on my file everything changes. They start to talk to my husband as if I can't make decisions for myself. Some don't even look me in the eye. It's as if they are frightened of catching some horrible disease.

The North-East London Foundation Trust (NELFT) Perinatal Parent Infant Mental Health Service is an integrated tier-three specialist multidisciplinary NHS service. I have run the 'Getting to Know You Group' in the team since 2010 and this chapter is based on the co-constructed experience of working with mothers and babies in the group over that period.

The context of the group

Run at a children's centre on a weekly slow open basis (not time limited), the group's simple aim is to help women feel less isolated and share experiences of becoming a mother. Women join then leave when things have improved, allowing new members to join at different stages. Potential group members find it helpful to hear that the group is only open to women referred to our service. They often assume that all the other mothers in the *regular* groups seem to be doing fine compared with them.

Most mothers referred, and often their partner, have a diagnosis of a serious mental illness. For others, the pregnancy or birth has triggered a puerperal psychosis or psychotic depression or a complex response to a traumatic birth. Most women in the group have concurrent psychiatric help from the service.

Multi-disciplinary discussions take place within the team. Working alongside social care and attending child protection meetings are a key part of the therapist's role, which helps hold the tension in assessing both parenting capacity and risk.

Babies, including antenatally, remain central in all discussions and are our patients in their own right with separate electronic case records from birth.

DOI: 10.4324/9781003310358-14

The getting-to-know-you group

- The group meets weekly for ninety minutes, with me as the sole conductor.
- I meet with mother and baby (and partner, if possible) for at least one session prior to joining the group.
- Mothers can join during pregnancy, usually in the third trimester or postnatally, and can stay until babies are about two years old.
- With no formal structured activity, all group members influence what gets talked about in the group. We all stay together for the entirety of the session.
- Spontaneous play in the session allows babies to express what cannot yet be put into words. Using a toy may be a baby's way of commenting about what is happening.
- Rules are different from adult therapy groups: women may have contact outside the group.
- As the only person who attends every session, I provide the consistency, keep the group themes alive and ensure absent members are kept in mind.
- Touching the babies is a common feature of the group as babies use not only their mother's body but also those of other members and the therapist. Adults do not touch each other.

Broadly speaking, the group is influenced by ideas from 'group analysis' and parent infant therapy. Change occurs at different levels, which Jones usefully categorises as:

> Firstly, the level of observable behaviours between baby and parent and what the behaviours mean; secondly, hypotheses about the influence of unconscious processes; and thirdly, the level of conscious narrative construction between therapist, parent/s and baby.
>
> (Jones, 2006, p. 301)

In adult work, past difficulties in relationships are largely reported in the present through the reconstruction of memory. In the Getting to Know You Group, we often have the opportunity to witness the difficulties in the mother-baby relationship in real time. The mother's difficulties and attachment style, and the potential for this to become the baby's developing attachment style, become evident as the difficulties unfold in the group.

What a group analyst brings to this kind of group is the training to hold in mind the complexity of the different sets of relationships in the group; to keep in mind the group process and themes over time and to work with unconscious processes, whether by putting these into words or not in the group. At times, the work takes place in the group analyst's mind.

Therapist flexibility – like a 'good enough' parent

Working clinically in this area requires an adaptation of any theoretical model, and usual boundaries in adult work are extended. The intimate nature of the work requires flexibility. In the group, I may hold babies at times or help wipe up sick. Around the time of the birth, we keep in touch by phone or I do home visits.

The work has a profound quality where we may witness a toddler taking their first steps or uttering first words. Strong real attachments form between babies and myself; these can help therapeutic change to occur quite quickly and the aim is to bring the baby's focus back to their mother.

The impact of working with risk

As therapists, we hear about disturbing fantasies in the mother's mind and help her make sense of these to avoid the risk of acting on these fantasies. In other settings, these can become concretised due to an anxiety about risk. The work in a multi-disciplinary team helps share this risk whilst holding psychiatric/psychotherapeutic tensions.

Working with babies activates intense feelings about how we were responded to ourselves as babies. These processes occur either consciously or unconsciously, and as professionals, we are not immune to them. To be put in touch as a professional with our own early baby self provides an opportunity to understand this better. Sometimes this can feel too raw and unwelcome, resulting in an urge to take action rather than think about the emotional experience, in order to tolerate uncertainty in the assessment of risk.

A community mental health nurse described her reaction after a home visit of a mother with a diagnosis of personality disorder who was struggling with her newborn baby: 'I was driving faster than usual and felt really wound up. A driver pushed in front of me suddenly and I wound down the window and swore at him. I never usually behave like that!' Team members in this field commonly report levels of rage that feel out of character, in identification with the dysregulated mother or baby, or feeling powerless, trapped and unable to move, in identification with the dependent baby. Feelings generated in the work are often akin to those a partner, mother, baby or grandmother might have.

Working with everyday concerns therapeutically

The group material is often focused on everyday aspects of parenting and experiences at different milestones in the babies' development. It can sound just like any other mother and baby group at times. With a more therapeutically oriented group, I respond to these concerns with subtlety, without using therapeutic jargon. The rationale is that the past is likely to repeat itself in the present, the repetition being linked to how the mother herself has been parented and her parents parented before her. This is explained by the metaphors of 'ghosts in the nursery' (Fraiberg et al., 1975) and 'angels in the nursery' (Lieberman et al., 2005). Increasing self-awareness can minimise the potential harm of repetition and allow babies to be freed from negative attributions. Encouraging mothers to show curiosity about the inner workings of the babies' minds can help improve parental 'reflective functioning' (Slade, 2005).

Often the process of change occurs when first both therapist and group members tune in to the mother's distress, giving space to recognise a feeling not yet acknowledged. Having the chance to express what is going on for her, the mother can begin to soften, and is then better able to respond to her baby.

Fear of Doing Damage – 'I swore I never would but I'm frightened that I am turning into my mother!' Dysregulation, confusion and isolation at the start of the group

A mother, Wanda, had presented to the service with a fear of becoming a bad mother. She had experienced inadequate parenting with sexual and physical abuse as a child and had a diagnosis of emotionally unstable personality disorder.

Wanda arrived late with her seven-month-old baby Milly, flustered and frustrated, cuddled her briefly, and then placed her in the circle at a distance from her. This was unusual. She looked visibly distressed. It was not clear why she kept her baby Milly at a distance. Was she seeking some relief from her demands or trying to protect her baby from her, allowing her daughter to have contact with another mother, whom she thought would do a better job?

Past and present collapse in the moment

Wanda described how Milly's bottle had been leaking so she had bought a new brand. Her baby had refused to feed from it this morning. She was struggling to wean Milly, even though she had been encouraged to start offering solids. She had felt criticised by health visitors for having a bottle that leaked. She said she felt ashamed as she had tried to be patient and could not understand why Milly would not take the milk like she usually did. Then she had 'lost it' and shouted at her. This had never happened before.

She started to cry. One of the other mothers was engaging baby Milly with a toy as she spoke. Wanda looked at me and said, 'I don't know what to do now'. I was in touch with her desperation and her longing and dependency on me to make it better by 'feeding her' with the right answer.

Aware of the mother's chronic compulsive eating problem, I suggested that something powerful had happened that morning that perhaps was not just about her daughter not taking the milk but maybe something connected with how she herself had been fed in her early life.

Reparative experience? – the same, or a different response?

Wanda then talked for the first time in the group about being forced when younger to eat food she did not like, until she gagged. She also remembered at other times feeling very hungry, as she was not fed regularly. She was horrified that she had become like her mother in shouting at Milly and hated herself for it. She looked at us sheepishly, as if she expected to be judged by the group, just as her family would have done.

The group does the work – sharing experiences with peers

Instead of judging, one mother talked about how difficult she had found it when her son had refused to drink from anything but one kind of bottle. She had been 'tearing her hair out not knowing what was wrong', and suggested Wanda change the teat of the old bottle rather than changing the bottle itself. She added that babies could be so powerful in rejecting food when something was wrong and how rejecting of the mother it could feel. I added my own thought that eating was the first thing we learned to control in life and refusal to eat was an early way of protesting when things just did not feel right.

Another mother talked about her own eating problems in the past and how she too had been forced to eat food that she did not like. She then went on to make a connection with her anxiety:

> When I was a compulsive eater I didn't know how to gauge when I was hungry or full. I guess that is why I struggle so much now with the feeding. It feels such a responsibility because they could die if they don't get enough!

A few mothers agreed and went on to share how difficult it was for them to give up breastfeeding or the bottle, when they had taken such pleasure in it, as they felt rejected as if they were not needed any more when their babies started to eat solids more independently.

Getting into the minds of the babies

Wanda insisted that Milly just was not ready to eat solid foods yet. She had tried during the week but her daughter had just spat the food out.

It transpired that she had given her porridge but had not added salt or sugar as they were bad for her. Someone responded gently, 'I don't blame her! It won't taste of anything! I usually mash up banana in mine'.

Babies help each other in the group

A fifteen-month-old boy, Joshua, went over to his mother. Sensing that he was hungry, she gave him a small snack. Milly looked towards her with interest. She checked with Wanda if it was okay for Milly to have some. Wanda hesitated but then agreed. Joshua's mother said, 'Shall we give Milly a bit?' Joshua moved towards Milly with his own piece in one hand and gave a bit to her with the other. Milly picked it up, smelled it, got it between her fingers with intense concentration then sucked it. The group was transfixed in silence, giving space and attention to her exploration. I encouraged Wanda to move closer so she could watch what was happening. Milly was clearly enjoying the new sensation, making appreciative noises. Wanda smiled, visibly moved, and was able to reflect on the difference between herself as a child and Milly. Milly was being uninhibited and allowed to explore with her own hands and at her own pace something she, Wanda, had never been allowed to do.

Separating out past from present

As the session progressed and we moved on to other things, Wanda was able to reclaim her baby and they had some moving, playful interactions. At the next session, Wanda told us that she had been enjoying experimenting, cooking new foods for Milly, and reported, 'She is learning what she wants in life!'

Reflection

Wanda felt misunderstood by the professionals' not recognising the roots of her difficulty, which left her feeling inadequate and confused about why she was struggling with something apparently so basic. She expected to be judged for her inadequacies not only by the professionals but also by the group, just as in her family.

In the group, we are repeatedly forced to witness distressing moments when a mother's response to her baby is less than adequate. This is difficult to bear at times but what is crucial is persevering with trying to understand the difficulty. If we can trust the group process, what unfolds over time is how the mother herself was mothered.

It often comes as a relief to have normalised a tendency to revert to saying the things that our mothers once said to us. We often hear, 'I couldn't help myself! It just came out of my mouth!' Feelings of guilt about inadequacies often get voiced in the group. Where there is a resistance to change over time, interventions to protect the baby from the potential damage do need to be considered. In cases where a mother has good intentions and a willingness to change, she can learn a lot from others in the group.

Rather than castigating themselves, the mothers are encouraged to think about the inevitability of ruptures in parenting and that what is crucial is the way in which ruptures can get repaired. Perhaps in all parenting, there is a tension between 'repetition compulsion' (Freud and Freud, 2001) and an opportunity through parenting to repair earlier experiences.

Babies as equal group members and contributors

This example demonstrates how babies are active and equal participants and their contributions crucial for the functioning of the group. The innocent forgiving gaze or longing of one baby often stirs maternal feelings in another mother unable to feel these feelings for her own baby. This is when a baby can offer something more powerful than any therapist.

Babies often initiate encounters, which are meaningful, as Milly and Joshua did in the example above. This helps mothers consider that they too may have been uninhibited at this age and that something has happened to make them less likely to trust and want to make social connections.

The long slow open nature of the group means that more experienced members, mothers and older babies alike, help the newer members develop, remembering what it was like when they were struggling, giving hope that if they stick at coming to the group, however difficult they find it, that it is possible that things can improve.

'Claiming the baby'

Many mothers find it hard to believe that they are the most important person in their baby's life. Through the group, they can begin to see that whilst their baby is capable of seeking out contact with a range of people, ultimately they will have a preference for mother (James, 2016).

One mother, who was planning to give her baby up for adoption, looked on as I engaged her baby and he smiled and babbled at me as I talked with him. The mother was convinced that he preferred me, just as she felt that her baby preferred her own mother. I told the mother that he was smiling at me because I was talking with him, and I spoke with the baby about how he was trying so hard to let his mother know how important she was to him but she was struggling to believe this. I encouraged the mother to practise chatting to him about everyday things and the following session she reported really enjoying the connection. Their relationship began to improve and she went on to keep him.

Change often occurs non-verbally through imitation and 'mirroring'. One mother's stroke of her baby's head finds its way travelling round the group, quite unconsciously. Often a deadness or isolation at the start of a session changes to something more alive and social. Both babies' and mothers' faces light up as in unspoken recognition, and multiple connections can get made. We create the conditions for Foulkes and Anthony's (1984) 'hall of mirrors' to happen, where each group member finds a range of mirrors in other group members to help discover who they are through both similarities and differences.

Thinking about disturbed feelings

Bringing a range of disturbance into the group can create an anxiety in the therapist about what we might be exposing mothers and babies to. Encouraging difficulties to be talked about freely can prove fruitful to the group's functioning. When one mother can take a risk, such as Wanda telling the group that she shouted at Milly and was on the verge of force-feeding her, others will usually follow, finding an opportunity to reveal their own untold fears.

Sharing the experience of being a mother can be a great leveller so that women from all walks of life from asylum seekers to high-powered professionals can help each other. Group dynamics of competition and envy can usually be put aside, in order to privilege the shared need for understanding and acceptance and the shame at not feeling good enough.

The potential for change in the group

Change is not always easy and not every mother can be helped to do an adequate job as a parent. The women in the example I have used were motivated to change, did not want to repeat their own childhood experience and had the potential to tune in to their babies' needs, with the help of the group. Due to the plasticity of babies' brains, problems in attachment have the potential to be resolved quite quickly. Helping each other, the mothers can grow in confidence and feel a sense that they matter. They often gain an awareness of their own authority as they develop more confidence in being a mother. They can start to translate this to groups outside and find it easier to function at work, in the family and in social situations.

Babies get to see others their own size, build confidence, and discover that they too have something to offer and some agency to have an impact on others. As younger babies join, older babies have to learn to be gentle, and to share and cooperate. They learn to use a group situation with peers, a life skill that can potentially compensate for difficult experiences at home or in relationships throughout their lives.

Acknowledgement

I am grateful to all the mothers and babies I have worked with who have taught me so much, not only about the work but also about myself.

Part 4

Gender and norms

Introduction

Gender and sexuality, both connected with norms, are topics both hotly debated in the public domain. Outmoded categories of gender and sex are being relinquished, and new ones are being defined. Psychotherapeutic schools of thought are following this trend. Denigrating prejudices and obsolete power privileges are no longer tolerated. Pathologising people for being different is no longer acceptable. Things are in flux and new attitudes regarding gender and norms are needed. We need to find new ways of talking, a new kind of language to discuss these issues and get hold of the new developments. Gender and norms are extremely important issues that affect people in their personal lives. Issues around these themes come up frequently in therapy groups and group members can get extremely engaged defending their personal views.

Several viewpoints are presented on how the topic of Gender and Norms can be understood and debated in the field of group analysis. The first three chapters in Part 4 are talking about the role of maternal and paternal qualities in group analytic theory by elucidating first the maternal quality of the matrix, second the conductor's role as father and third proposing a new term 'patrix' to initiate a group analytic theory of leadership. In contrast to these viewpoints, the following chapter elucidates the authority that lies in the group-as-a-whole rather than in the hands of the group conductor. In counterbalance to the power of the conductor, the authority that lies in the group itself is illuminated as the democratic hallmark of group analysis. It is defined and named as 'normative' authority.

Amélie Noack suggests in the first chapter that the group analytic concept 'matrix' needs to be further differentiated to get hold of processes within the matrix. She suggests a new way to understand the concept of the matrix by differentiating it into a structural and a dynamic component, so that the matrix as a container can be appraised as separate from the transformative processes occurring within this container.

DOI: 10.4324/9781003310358-15

David Vincent looks in the second chapter at the impact of gender and the father's role. He describes being a man in his role of conductor and how the group used him as a man, what they did to him as a person and how that affected him personally. He wonders how gender manifests in the group and how a woman would be affected by these dynamics and explores the father's role in connection with the arrival of a new baby or new group member. The 'instruction of the father' based on the Bible is compared and contrasted with 'the law of thy mother', considering all this from the perspective of the group-analyst-in-the-group.

Amélie Noack attempts to initiate the development of a group analytic theory of leadership by complementing 'matrix' with the concept of 'patrix'. The 'patrix', denoting the group conductor's qualities relating to their use of authority and power in their interaction with the group, evokes in the interaction with the structure of the matrix the group analytic processes of 'ego training in action'. The directive, but benign and thoughtful activity of the patrix, she suggests, would be a particularly useful concept for female group conductors.

Sarah Tucker introduces the concept of normative authority, contrasting it with the 'patrix' and Freud's idea of the Super-ego. Normative authority highlights the democratic hallmark of group analysis, namely that authority lies in the group-as-a-whole rather than just in the hands of the group conductor. This means taking the group analytic premise of the priority of the group seriously in contrast to the role of the conductor. She illustrates her understanding with examples and tests her view against Nitsun's notion of the anti-group. Her argument points to the fact that the relationship between the conductor's authority and normative authority in the group should be able to withstand social destructive forces.

Chapter 11

The matrix as container and crucible

Amélie Noack

Introduction

The term 'matrix' is an important term in group analysis. According to Foulkes (1986), matrix describes a network or medium, formed by the members of the group, which as a web of communications is also having an effect on the members of the group and forming them in turn. Each and every member of the group represents a nodal points in this matrix.

Example

A patient in one of my groups provided a spontaneous example for this experience, when he said six months into the group's life:

> It's amazing! We come here together from all different backgrounds with so many different experiences and it all somehow comes together in the group. The group is really important to me. I feel better afterwards and wait for the next session.

Parallel to his words, he was bending forward and holding his hands into the space of the group, moving them in and out, as if knitting various strands together. This communication, derived from his felt experience, held a power of conviction for his fellow group members, which none ever so clever interpretation by me could have matched. His communication evoked a moment of resonance in the group and people began to describe how they each had made their original commitment to the group. This initiated a criss-crossing pattern of interactions, indicating the establishment of the holding matrix. Both James (1982a) and Powell (1989) observe that the container function of the matrix starts to function fully, when the movement of interactions in the group displays a criss-crossing pattern going through the centre of the circle of the group with the interactions 'flying out in all directions' (James, 1982).

DOI: 10.4324/9781003310358-16

The matrix – various theoretical approaches

The theory on the matrix has been developed by a number of eminent group analysts (James, 1982; Powell, 1989, 1991a; Prodgers, 1990; Zinkin, 1989). This chapter reflects on these earlier works and suggests that the matrix needs to be differentiated into a structural and dynamic aspect. The first aspect of the matrix, designating the container function, is described as a precondition for the second, that is the dynamic and transformative processes occurring within this container, since only when the matrix functions as a container can the process matrix come into being. The differences between the structure and the dynamics of the matrix are then elucidated in application to groups through concepts derived from alchemy, the mediaeval forerunner of both chemistry and psychology.

Following Foulkes, James (1982) highlights in his paper the connection between the matrix and Bion's container concept as a structure that holds and contains, and Winnicott's transitional space, an area of transformation and development. He describes the two most important qualities of the matrix as first providing a holding and containing environment and second a space in which change and development can occur.

Prodgers (1990) returns to Foulkes' association of matrix with mother. Matrix is Latin for womb or uterus, the place where new life starts. He describes the dual nature of the group as mother based on Jungian theory in reference to the archetype of the Great Mother. The two different aspects of the Great Mother and therefore of the group are first her holding and nurturing aspect and second her terrifying and engulfing aspect. These two facets, Prodgers suggest, need to be integrated through a process called 'coniunctio'. The experience of wholeness arises out of the integration of contradictory feelings such as joy and despair, love and hate or good and evil and is called the 'conjunction of opposites'.

Powell (1989, 1991, 1993), a group analyst and Jungian analyst, develops his ideas of the matrix in relation to the 'new physics' by drawing on relativity theory, the principle of connectedness and the wave/particle duality of the quantum field. His idea of a 'relativity' matrix highlights the generative function of mind in creating three-dimensional reality and he describes the wave/particle quantum effect as reflected in the experience of fusion and separateness between group members. Just as solid matter and space are confluent, he says, so are mind and body. Therapist and group members might all be thoroughly immersed in each other's electromagnetic fields, with lines of force conceived as passing right through the individual members, comparable to a magnetic field. This view would imply a new meaning of the term 'projection', since it would explain the phenomenon that a group member may express an insight of the conductor, if the conductor can hold it in mind without verbalising it. "The 'new physics'", Powell (1992) says, "makes it plain that we exist in, and are part of, a matrix of awesome energy". He concludes that themes like relativity, wave/particle duality and connectedness, and their integration into a cosmological whole, are all represented within the mandala – the circle – of the group.

Zinkin (1989) quotes Jung as referring to the unconscious as "the matrix of the human mind and its inventions" and applies this to the group as a representation of the self:

> The group-self ... provides the group members with some notion of a larger transcendent self, ultimately a sense of 'all there is', ... as being undivided, and ... this is a religious experience.
>
> (Zinkin, 1989, p. 213)

The self – and in analogy the group – represents something sacred or spiritual. The sacred space of the group – Zinkin reiterates Powell here – can be considered akin to a mandala, an image of sacred space and the circle of chairs designates this. Each mandala has its own motif, usually based on the squaring of the circle in the form of a cross, a 'quaternio' or foursome, signifying an image of wholeness. Interestingly, Foulkes thought that the ideal group was also made up of a 'quaternio', seven patients plus the conductor, making eight people altogether.

All the above perspectives describe the matrix predominantly as a container and a description of the dynamic processes occurring 'within' this matrix is neglected.

Towards a dynamic interpretation of the matrix

A paradigm shift in the direction of thinking about processes in application to the concept of the matrix was already suggested by Ralph Stacey (2000). Powell (1991) and Zinkin (1989) refer in their above-mentioned papers also to a connection between the term 'matrix' and the alchemical vessel, which was also called matrix. In both these matrices, powerful transformative processes can take place.

The alchemical metaphor

Most people have heard about alchemy only as the dubious attempt to turn lead into gold and do not know that scientists, like Newton or Paracelsus studied alchemy. In actual fact, our scientific attitude today goes back to the alchemists' emphasis on the combination of both theory and practice. It was essential for them to both contemplate their work 'and' to experiment to substantiate their thinking. Medieval Alchemy therefore has in addition to its experimental side a psychological component. Specific terms, still applied in chemistry today, but also found in the current psychoanalytical vocabulary, portray this connection, and processes like sublimatio, fixatio, separatio or condensatio were originally names for specific alchemical operations.

Jung (1974), working as a psychiatrist with psychotic patients, got interested in the psychological interpretation of the seemingly bizarre imagery of alchemy, when he found that the insights of the alchemists' into their mental and emotional processes during their experiments in the laboratory showed similarities with the symptoms of his psychotic patients. Psychology as a science only developed in the 19th century and Jung (1974) realised that the alchemists watched and studied in the alchemical retort or 'matrix' their own psychological processes in projection onto the enigmatic conjunction of elements (Jung, 1955, p. 460). The thoughts and feelings about the transformations the alchemists observed in their retorts provided Jung with a way to understand and treat mental disturbances, especially psychotic processes.

The analogy between group analysis and alchemy is based on the fact that in both, group analysis and alchemy, various elements or ingredients react with each other within a container. In the group, this is represented by the circle of chairs and the various personalities of the group members, the space within the group reflecting the alchemists' laboratory.

The matrix as container and crucible

Foulkes' equation of matrix and group needs to be examined further. The group is not the matrix, the group is a collection of people. The matrix is a conceptual abstraction.

The holding matrix

The circular setting of a groups together with the boundaries of time and space can also be perceived as a vessel or container. To hold this space and its boundary securely is essential for group analysis. The alchemical vessel or crucible had similar significance for the alchemists. It needed to be a solid and sound container and had to be securely closed or 'hermetically' sealed in order to hold and survive the explosive and corrosive processes of the work. Hermes, the guardian spirit of alchemy, provided the name for the secure sealing of the alchemical vessel. Similar to the hermetic seal of the alchemists, any leakage from the group or a breaking of boundaries, like outside contact between group members, can pose a real threat to the work.

Time, space and the circle of chairs of the group visually mark the holding matrix, and in group analytic terms include an understanding of the importance of confidentiality and boundaries, shared by the group-as-a-whole. As soon as the holding matrix is established, akin to 'hermetically' sealing the alchemical vessel, the preconditions for change are given. Now the holding matrix serves as a secure container – the group has become a group.

The process matrix

The alchemists devoted a major part of their work to the observations of the processes within the alchemical vessel. They scrutinised the rising vapours, which indicated one of the most important processes in the alchemical opus, called sublimation, and they examined the condensation of liquids. In a similar way, observation and analysis of the dynamic and transformative processes within the central space of the group are possible. Through catching sight of unconscious phenomena in this space, the process matrix can become virtually visible. Foulkes seemed to suggest something similar when he said:

> It would be quite impossible (for the therapist) to follow each individual at the same time. He focuses on the **total interactional field, on the matrix** [my emphasis] in which these unconscious reactions meet.
>
> (Foulkes and Anthony, 1957)

The idea of applying insights from alchemy to groups arose originally when I observed a virtual circle of flames on the table in the middle of a group at the moment, when a group member, a devoted nun and sworn to celibacy, shared her experience of falling passionately in love.

Dynamic processes of transformation

The developmental journey of a group can be compared to the transformations that occur in alchemy, starting with an unstable, brittle and possibly fragmented state – symbolised by the alchemical lead – to eventually arrive at a stable, coherent and reliable state – the alchemists' gold. It is a process that moves through specific stages of transformation, each with their particular images and qualities, which, in turn, relate to specific emotional experiences or particular feeling states. The basic alchemical model has three stages, corresponding to the colours black, white and red.

The first stage: Nigredo – baptism by fire

The first stage of the alchemical process is called Nigredo, which is Latin for blackness. It is a stage of darkness and despair, where things are chaotic and confused. As the original stage of primal chaos, it is symbolised by the alchemical element of lead.

The alchemists used to heat the alchemical vessel and its content in order to promote change and the Nigredo can feel extremely hot. Through heat, the original substances in the crucible are broken down until they crumble to ashes and dust. This parallels the rise of the emotional temperature in a therapy group when change is imminent. Emotional turbulence accompanies the breaking down of old psychic structures in an individual or the group-as-a-whole. This is a frightening, possibly terrifying experience, because old defences may be gone but the new psychic organisation has not yet come into being. Expressions like 'I feel totally lost', 'I'm falling apart' or 'I feel in bits' may allude to the Nigredo. In this situation, empathy is needed, and if the group is not able to provide this, the conductor will have to make sure everybody feels held and understood. Working through the Nigredo can take a long time. It is extremely hard to tolerate unbearable annihilation anxieties and endure feelings of pain, loss, abandonment and despair.

The whole group may be in a state of 'black' and 'heavy' depression. People who would have preferred individual therapy, now express resentment about being in the group and having to fight the confusion of becoming mixed up with others. The Nigredo often re-occurs before or after a break or when someone joins or leaves the group, because the loss of the old situation needs mourning and working through.

Example

Shortly before the Easter break everybody in the group was talking about feeling suicidal. In the heavy atmosphere, the space within the group seemed like a 'black pit'. I pointed out that the coming break may be looming like an unbridgeable gap. Suddenly, one group member took his sunglasses out, telling us they were glasses for the most intense sunlight and that he wanted them as a protection against the glaring ceiling lights. Others pointed out that they could not see his eyes anymore and he took them off again. Another group member tried the glasses and when she found she could hardly see anything through them – started to giggle. The atmosphere in the group changed. The combination between glaring light and complete blackness resembled the 'sol niger', Latin for 'black sun', the alchemical name for an eclipse of the sun and another image for the Nigredo. It also constituted a 'coniunctio', a coming together of opposites, despair and laughter, which produced an emotional shift.

The second stage: Albedo – immersion in the bath

At the end of the Nigredo, dust and ashes are left in the alchemical retort and water or other solvents would be added to these sediments to initiate the second alchemical stage, called the Albedo, which is Latin for whiteness.

Psychologically speaking, empathy is needed to initiate the Albedo. A liquid binding agent in the form of tears, sorrow, sweat or grief is added to the dust left by the Nigredo. Defences against pain, sorrow and grief are melting and the dregs of the old psychic state are washed away by the watery flow of emotion. Groups are often deeply moved by each other's suffering, courage and pain. To the mixture of empathy and compassion, mutual understanding and the milk of human kindness (Noack, 2002a) are added and start to create a new cohesion. Experiences of mutuality and reciprocity develop in the group and gradually mature into an increasing awareness of interdependence.

Example

Hannah complained about her husband's jealousy. When John interrupted her continuously, she got angry. The group suggested they should give each other more space and the atmosphere relaxed. Katja then mentioned how difficult it is for children to move from single letters to connected writing and Harry remembered that he felt so ashamed about this that he stopped going to school. He hid in his room and felt an outcast. "You must have felt imprisoned and locked in", the group suggested. Another group member shared that her mother used to lock her out at the same age. "You would have needed a mother to **be** there for you, not an overpowering mother!" was the empathic response. Harry broke out in tears, then looked around the group and said in an amazed tone: "I can't believe it, you **do** understand!"

This example demonstrates mutual empathy and understanding between group members. It also shows, the interplay of opposites, an important characteristic of the Albedo, when speaking is interrupted, single letters cannot be connected and children are locked in or locked out. In this interplay of opposites, empathy alternates with envy, and there is increasingly a letting go, with a final release of tears. The Albedo is a watery state and expressions like 'being at sea', 'going under' or 'being in a fog' belong here, as does anything 'wet' including sexuality or feelings of shame and guilt. Empathy and challenge are both needed to move the process on.

The third stage: Rubedo – the philosopher's stone

The dawning of the third stage of the Rubedo is symbolised by the image of the reddish golden colour of the rising sun. In this final stage, the interplay of opposites has ended and the opposites are coming together on a new level, symbolising new life and birth. This final stage has new qualities, it is stable and reliable. Its symbols are the philosopher's stone, indicating solidity and durability, or the alchemists' gold, signifying something valuable and shiny.

In the Rubedo emerges a new sense of self, based on the awareness of an ego in interdependence with and in relation to a greater unit. For a group, this means an awareness of mutuality through the understanding that an individual and its group are always located in reciprocal relation to each other. 'Group' may now also stand for a greater unit, represented by one's family, one's community or even one's culture, and can also extend to life or the universe as a whole. The new sense of a self in relation to the world at large is accompanied by new mental clarity and distinction, akin to the alchemist's gold, and a capacity for comprehension which is solid, coherent and reliable, like the philosopher's stone. With this new perspective, it becomes possible to make diligent choices and to take responsibility for the consequences of one's own actions, since the challenges of the transformational processes of life do not provoke the same levels of anxiety as before.

Example

For a couple of weeks, the group had worked very quietly and consistently at a new level of psychological depth, when Tom put this new experience into words on behalf of everybody, by saying: "It has taken me a long time to understand how the group really works. I also benefit when others talk about something and my comments are useful in a different way for each of us". A group member replied, "Yes, it's not about getting your fifteen minutes, as you thought at the beginning". Everybody laughed. This was a precious experience, especially since the group knew that in the next week, a new member would be joining the group. They knew from experience that this would not be easy and would bring new difficulties.

This example illustrates that the Rubedo is a fleeting experience, short and sweet. After the exquisite moment of insight or understanding, new difficulties will arise and new challenges and struggles will have to be faced. The process commences again.

The matrix and alchemy: processes of becoming

Each alchemical stage, Nigredo, Albedo or Rubedo, describes a distinctive emotional experience or complex feeling-state, which, in turn, can be located within a developmental process. Being able to locate a group's emotional communication within this process can give the conductor options to intervene in stage-appropriate ways.

The holding matrix and the process matrix are both present at any given time. In parallel to the particle/wave-uncertainty in quantum mechanics, the matrix displays either the structural particle-nature of the container or the dynamic wave-nature of the process, depending on the focus of the conductor. In a newly established group, the conductor will probably focus mostly on the container aspect and shift the attention to the process matrix later. In an established group, the conductor will have to move from one to the other many times within one session.

The process matrix is that aspect of the matrix that is always in the process of becoming, which is in accordance with Stacey's view (2000) that

> [The] matrix as a network … self-organises to produce emergent patterns in its own evolution – in other words the matrix is forming itself.
>
> (Stacey, 2000, p. 501)

Since the matrix is

> not the result of a prior design or the revealing of an already existing, hidden whole. The authentic, absent whole is in the parts and emerges from the parts.
>
> (ibid., p. 506)

The process matrix is identical with this authentic, absent whole, which is always emergent. Like the transformations in alchemy, which are not the result of a prior design, but emerge in the course of the work from the constituent parts as a result of their combination, group analysis is never complete, but weaves forwards and backwards. It is creation always in the process of becoming. The matrix in its combination of container and process is not a thing or an object. It is what Stacey calls a no-thing or absent whole, "in the sense that we cannot grasp the whole" (Stacey, 2000, p. 506). While we may never be able to grasp the whole, we may well be able to observe it in its process of becoming. This is what group analysts do when they scan their groups, like alchemists gazing into their crucibles.

Chapter 12

The father in the group

David Vincent

Father and child

In Samuel Beckett's play 'Endgame', there are continuous references to fathers, and to injury (Beckett, 1958). The central character Hamm, who is blind and cannot walk, occupies a movable chair at the centre of the stage for the whole play, and he treats his servant Clov harshly. Clov, who can stand but cannot sit down, seems to have come to serve Hamm as a small boy and does not remember his father. Hamm's parents, Nagg and Nell, live in two dustbins at the front of the stage. They both lost their legs in a bicycling accident on their tandem. Everyone in the play is in some way injured or disabled. Even the toy dog that Hamm enjoys is missing a leg. Hamm feeds his parents on dog-biscuits and hates them, particularly his father for giving birth to him. He mocks them for this and for their injuries. "Accursed Fornicator! How are your stumps?" he says to Nagg early in the play. Later Hamm orders Clov to wake his father up and Nagg sits up from inside his dustbin. "I'm listening", he says. Hamm replies: "Scoundrel! Why did you engender me?". This is of course a good question and Nagg gives a brilliant answer: "I didn't know…that it'd be you" (ibid., p. 49).

Parents never know who their children will be; however, a strong relationship develops while the child is in the womb. Mothers and sometimes fathers draw complex conclusions about the future from the baby's behaviour in utero. The baby kicks strongly, for example, and so will turn out to be a marvellous footballer, or the baby is quiet and passive and therefore will be good-natured. The rich emotional family life of pregnancy is full of both, imaginings and fears for the future, and it is not too big a leap to think that something similar happens to a psychotherapy group and its group analyst when a new patient is expected. The new patient's arrival, for example, always rouses up, in every group, some of the sort of feelings that arise in a family on the birth of a new sibling: joy, rage, hope, rivalry and envy.

What they don't know is what sort of person has joined them. Like the parents and siblings of a new baby, they may have a mixture of fears, hopes and expectations. They may be determined, consciously and unconsciously,

DOI: 10.4324/9781003310358-17

to shape the new patient or baby in ways that will suit them or in ways that they think may be helpful and protective. In a group, established patients may make a point of protecting the other group members, particularly from the group analyst. They may warn the new member not to take too much notice of them. One long lasting group used to say to me: "there you go again, spoiling things. Everything was going well until you said that." Once, rather naively, I said to them, in an attempt at explanation, that I was trying to be a group analyst. After a furrowed-brow sort of silence, once of them said wearily: "well, you are very trying." This was, of course, contemptuous, but it was also defensive, perhaps the interpretation that had annoyed them had been right. At least it was a good sign that I was getting under the skin of the group, disturbing their complacency. This particular group, like many others, loved the group but hated the analysis.

The new baby, the new group member and the process of socialisation

A new patient, like a child in the family, often takes their cue from the group. Some of this guidance is helpful and liberating and some is not. The group socialises its new members into the way that the group does things, and this is of course not always either welcome or helpful. One of the most difficult things for a group analyst is to understand, and work with, this socialising process. At the same time, the group is sometimes helpful and right. For a new patient to be socialised into a new way of being with people can in itself be transformative, both for the new patient and the established group. This is particularly true for patients who have been, as it were, over-socialised into a rigid family or a religious or political group or who are, for whatever reason, excessively self-critical. This also includes those who have had a lot of contact with medical and psychiatric services, and who have become socialised into being that sort of patient. Joining a group with other suffering people, who talk very openly to one another, and in a very challenging way to the group analyst, may in itself be liberating. A new patient arrived in the group in a rage with her psychiatrist because he had recently told her that he was referring her to group therapy, and in addition, that she had a borderline personality disorder. After a brief silence, a long-serving patient with a rich and complex illness history leaned forward, tapped her on the knee, and said: "Don't worry, dear. I've got one of those."

So, the group, like the family, takes on the challenge of changing and being changed by the new patient, like the family by the new baby. This is an exciting and life-enhancing process, accompanied by grief, envy and rage, as the group members settle down into their family and sibling roles. Each group member has a rigid set of relationships and taken-for-granted ways of relating in their mind, their original internalised group, which they then try to foist on the rest of the group in the present moment. The group, together and individually, resist this process. At the same time, each of the members is doing the same thing. This process continues through interchanging sets of connections in the group, usually through a constantly changing and evolving movement between two-person and three-person relationships, as I have argued elsewhere (Vincent, 2016, p. 128).

The 'group-analyst-in-the-group'

This chapter is concerned with the role of the father in group analysis and the father appears in various forms, as tyrant, tormentor, lover, abuser, companion and co-conspirator, in many of the two- and three-person relationships in the group. The group of course has the ability to make anyone in the group, patient or analyst, in the moment into whoever the group want them or needs them to be. This movement between imagination and reality and the experience, in the imaginative phase, of the feeling of a 'group mind' and of a shared reconstruction of reality, runs alongside the movement between two and three-person relations. It is only momentary, and indeed there is an argument that the group, as a group, only really exists in the present moment and then is instantly lost into the demands of individual reality as things move on.

What this can mean is that the 'father in the group' is usually, but not necessarily, a man. At times, the group so badly needs to work on their relationships with men and fathers that in the absence of a suitable man they have to make a new father in the group, whether it is a woman patient, a woman group analyst or a composite figure cobbled together, to allow them to do their work. And if the group is working together well, then this is just what happens, and it goes away immediately the work is done. This would be a clear example of the 'group-analyst-in-the-group', where the group members as individuals clearly see that their group analyst is a woman, but in order for the group to do its analytic work, the group unconsciously creates out of and alongside their individual group analyst this complex composite object: the 'group-analyst-in-the group'. This is not a shared psychotic fantasy or a 'regression', as Bion (1961) would have it, but is a brief moment of necessary shared imaginative capacity in the group. Momentarily the group together create and reconstruct the group analyst, in conjunction with the group, into exactly the sort of object that they all need to do their work: the 'group-analyst-in-the-group'.

So where does this leave the man, the group analyst, who is being even if only for a moment turned into a mother or a maternal 'group-analyst-in-the-group', or the woman who is being turned into a father or the composite object? The immediate counter-transference sensations may be interesting, disconcerting or disturbing, and the group analyst might feel intruded upon and controlled. In itself this might be useful information about the individual members of the group and their experience of growing up in their 'original group'.

"Throw off the numbing feeling of reality", says Bion (1961, p. 149) in advising the working group psychotherapist. In other words, don't let yourself as the group analyst be controlled and driven by what is actually probably a taken-for-granted 'un-thought' state of mind, a reaction to a 'Basic Assumption' in the group (Bion, 1961). In the moment that is easier said than done, when the group analyst is in the middle of being transformed into the group's needed object: a 'group-analyst-in-the-group'. The group's imaginative reconstruction of the group analyst's mind, body and gender may, however brief, be experienced as a seduction or a violation and attack and the group analyst may feel guilty, wounded and vulnerable.

The father in the group: A necessary evil?

We are concerned here with the father in the group. I have been arguing for the transformative power of the group, imaginatively working together, to recreate their necessary object in whatever form they need. This need may result in the group turning a male group analyst into a primarily female group-analyst-in-the-group, or indeed into a combined male and female object. Does something similar to this happen to a woman group analyst, at the same point in the group? I can only give an account of how this all feels, and what it means, to a male group analyst, and how that connects to the role of the Father in the group. After all, to quote Stephen Daedalus, from 'Ulysses' by James Joyce: "A father, Stephen said, battling against hopelessness, is a necessary evil" (Joyce, 1922/1960, pp. 265–266). In other words, a group is always a family with a mother and a father, and an all-male group with a male group analyst always creates or behaves as though it has created a mother in the group, in whatever form, saintly or devilish, that the group needs at that point. Sometimes the group needs a mother and sometimes a father, and if one isn't there, they will therefore create them, even if only for a moment.

How does a male group analyst step outside his maleness and fatherhood? He has a male body, which he is used to, and is part of what may be a continuing male lineage. It is a considerable psychic task to step outside the demands of the lineage of the Y-chromosome. But group analysts have to be able to find a way of imagining, and then triangulating. In the group, if nowhere else, a male group analyst has to be able at times to stand outside his maleness (and fatherhood) to see if he can work out what is happening around him in the group, and then assess how much of it is to do with him being and behaving (whatever, in the moment, that consists of) like a man and a father and what effect that is having on the group-as-a-whole and the individual group members. I assume that a similar dilemma affects woman group analysts.

Now, one way of doing this, that helps us all, is to trust the group. This is, however, always easier said than done, and it has to be an active decision on a moment-by-moment basis. After all, the group is usually more robust than its group analyst and often, as a whole, more thoughtful and imaginative than he, if we go along with Foulkes' maxim that the group 'collectively constitutes the norm from which the individuals deviate' (Foulkes, 1948). This, my experience tells me, is not only useful but true, although if I am at that moment in the group in an anxious counter-transference state of mind, it seems completely counter-intuitive. Which is why, in my view, groups that are run without the benefit of group-analytic practice, particularly these three linked central concepts of trusting the group, the matrix and Foulkes' maxim, often founder and sink into despair, fruitless disputes or continuous grinding interpretations of the negative transference.

If we can remind ourselves to trust the group to get on with it around us to do their work, unimpeded by our anxiety, then we can occasionally have, if only briefly, the privileged experience of seeing ourselves being seen as part of the group-analyst-in-the-group, just as the group sees us, and it is often a strange almost uncanny experience. Now in particular, we can sometimes see, if we are lucky, the most hard-to-reach, taken-for-granted aspects of ourselves, which to others primarily or most obviously perhaps consist in our gender. I don't want to over-simplify this. Dependent entirely on where I am and who I am with, others looking at me might see first a man, a white man, an old man or a middle-class man. In my group, they might see all, or any, or none of these, as well as 'the group-analyst-in-the-group', a mother and/or a father, a child, a sibling, a tyrant, a lover, a ghost, a persecutor or someone to be manipulated, punished, seduced or ignored. In the group unconscious we are infinitely malleable.

The group, if they are working together over time on something important for them all, then they might construct this capacious new composite object, the group-analyst-in-the-group out of parts of themselves and the group analyst. This object lasts only a moment in time as it is an unconscious group process. The group analyst feels for that moment that he or she is being transformed, broken up and reassembled into the composite object, along with others or parts of others from the group. It is therefore a group-specific countertransference phenomenon, and it is important to emphasise that this is specifically a help-seeking movement in the group. A newly formed object is needed in the group's attempt to both understand and to change. It is neither defensive nor an attack on the group analyst, and it therefore does not rouse up fear, anger or existential anxiety in the group analyst, although the counter-transference may include confusion, dizziness, disorientation and a curiously pleasant feeling of being lost and far from home. It is very brief, as it is only in the present moment.

As well, we are implicitly and sometimes explicitly, if we or the group see it and comment on it, being involved in the business of mirroring in the group, and we have our own self being continually reflected or distorted back to us (Pines, 1982). If I look in a mirror, I do not see myself, of course, as others see me, because of lateral distortion. Perhaps I am never just me, being reflected back to myself in the group, but rather, at times, this composite figure of the group-analyst-in-the-group. In other words, we have all the ordinary complexities of how we don't know we are seen or how we are being experienced at any one moment in time in relation to others, plus the extraordinarily interesting richness and confusion of being this odd composite figure of the group-analyst-in-the-group. In the group, we are no longer who we thought we were outside the door of the group room. Once we close the door behind us we are something else, both a member and not a member, part of and separate from the group, available to be projected into, introjected, identified with, blamed, loved, hated, feared and persecuted.

The group process

What makes group analysis so interesting and so hard to follow is that all of the above can be going on in any one moment and in different combinations: loved by one, hated by two others, experienced as a loving father by the men or the women, and as a patriarchal tyrant by the men or the women, feared by the younger people, patronised by the older members. These are familiar feelings to group analysts.

We make ourselves available for this in the matrix as the group analyst and in this odd role as group-analyst-in-the-group, and we gradually get a grip on it, if we are lucky using our group analyst's tool kit. This consists of two major elements. First, our theoretical knowledge about how groups work, theory and technique, and our understanding of the individual patients, their history and character, and second, our subjective knowledge of what is happening in the moment through our counter-transference and our reverie.

How does this throw light on the father in the group? First, it is necessary to think about being brought up against this sudden realisation of how others see me in the group, particularly as a man and a father, and being made aware of how they then use me in the group. I will give three very straightforward examples from NHS groups several years ago. They highlight in particular how the group and individuals in the group deal with the problems that can arise from being a male therapist to female patients, particularly to women who have been abused by men. In general terms, I always find it helpful to remind myself that child sexual abuse is always a three-person or three-object problem. The most common version of this that we come across in our patients is a young adolescent girl abused by a step-father alongside the unconscious collusion or blindness of the mother. A victim, an abuser and a third who knows and does nothing.

These triangle of abuse dynamics are universal and take many forms, and all psychotherapists know that in the session, group or individual, the triangle gets repeated and moves about continuously. In a group, a patient may speak about their abuse as a victim and immediately the group analyst, group members, sub-groups or the group as a whole, volunteer for or get recruited into one of these three roles, and then it can switch about very rapidly. We all know that bewildering feeling of suddenly, while we thought we were listening attentively and with empathy, being treated with anger or hurt or contempt by the patient or other members of the group, as though we were the abuser or the one who knew and did nothing. I do not actually know if this is more difficult for male psychotherapists treating women victims of sexual abuse or assault by men. On the basis of initial assessments over many years, male and female victims of both family and stranger sexual abuse will often ask to see a female therapist for treatment. I think that this matters less in the long run for group treatment, perhaps because both abused male and female patients can find common cause with other abused patients, usually women, and together they can stand up to the men. If the group analyst is a man, this can be particularly helpful, although difficult for the group analyst.

Examples

The mature group can make you into what they need you to be at any one moment and sometimes this is surprisingly direct. In one group, there was a middle-aged woman from Malaysia, a devout Catholic who had been a nun when she was young. Hers was a touching story that the group enjoyed. She had joined a convent whose novices and young nuns worked as servants to priests and seminarians. She was assigned to a seminary for priests with a late-life vocation, so they were all older men who had led an ordinary life out in the world for many years. As a result, they expected to chat in a friendly way to the servant nuns when they were working, and the nuns responded. The superiors of the order found out and forbade the nuns to ever speak to the priests. My patient found this so unreasonable that she decided to leave the order. She led a difficult life, had unsuccessful relationships with men, which led to a daughter, and became depressed. She was very cautious and unresponsive in the group and particularly with me, avoiding any kind of intimacy. One day, the group tackled her and asked her about her relationships in the past and if she wanted one now. Very angrily, she said that she did not and that if anyone tried to get close to her, she would always "chop it off", making a cutting gesture with one hand onto the palm of the other hand, and glaring defiantly round the group.

In another group, the women were talking very critically about men and how awful they were. One woman, who was also always very cautious with me, said very dismissively that "men are just boys with money". I then pointed out that I was a man, sitting here in the group. Indignantly this patient pointed vigorously across the room and said in a loud voice "Well, you can leave that at the door".

The third example of these rather basic ways of dealing with the maleness and also, surely, the fatherliness of the male therapist is more painful. A woman, who was in the group for a long time, had grown up in great poverty with a crushed mother and a perverse father. They all lived and slept in one room. The father insisted on having often violent sex in front of my patient, when they were all in bed. Later she had got into a loving, but difficult relationship. She became a very devout Anglican and talked movingly in one group, about the struggle she often went through when praying to Christ on the cross, imagining and hating the thought that Christ had genitals, and dealing with this by negatively hallucinating them. She then looked at me and said that was the only way that she could tolerate me too, by hallucinating my genitals away.

I give these three rather straightforward examples, because they show very clearly how patients in the group can make of you what they will or what they need. In the unconscious, of course, body parts are infinitely interchangeable. The group will want you sometimes as a man and sometimes as a woman irrespective of what you actually are. Similarly, the group will make you sometimes a father and sometimes a mother, or neither. When I worked in a Drug Addiction Clinic, one day my trouser turn-up fell and I, pragmatically, fixed it with a staple. I then forgot about it and probably wore the trousers for a while with the staple in them. Some months later, a very hard-nosed, cynical, criminal heroin addict found out by chance that I was married, with children. He was astounded and told me that the staple in my turn-up a few months ago had suggested to him that I had no-none looking after me. I did not therefore have a family and was instead devoted in a monk-like way to the care only of my patients. He needed me not to be a father to anyone else except to him and the other patients of the clinic.

The necessary father

If we agree with Stephen Daedalus that a father is a necessary evil, and that therefore every group has one or needs one and will create one in their absence, where does this leave our understanding of the symbolic value of the father in the group? If we accept the malleability and flexibility of sexual and parental roles in the group unconscious, then what is it about these roles, particularly that of the father, that makes it desirable or undesirable at any one moment?

Let us start at the beginning, with the Old Testament and the Buddha. In the Old Testament, in *Proverbs*, it is said:

> 8. My Son, hear the instruction of thy father and forsake not the law of thy mother.
> 9. For they shall be an ornament of grace unto thy head and chains about thy neck.
>
> (Holy Bible, Proverbs 1.8 & 12.9, p. 551)

And the Buddha:

> A son can never show sufficient gratitude to his parents for their loving kindness, even were he to carry his father on his right shoulder and his mother on his left shoulder for 100 long years.
>
> (Lulu (trans), 1987, p. 40)

This is complicated, of course, and in one sense we know what the Buddha meant, and we can continually see in our groups, that even patients who have had a difficult and cruel childhood can sometimes become reconciled with and grateful to their depriving parents, not for their behaviour, but through a process of understanding how loss and trauma pass through the generations. It can be seen as an expression of the 'compulsion to repeat'.

At a CAMS Clinic, in a group of troubled parents of very unwell children, the mothers all agreed that they had, when young, formed a firm resolution not to be like their mothers and then found themselves doing exactly the same thing to their children as their mothers had done to them. But they acknowledged this together in the group and it was extremely moving. As they mirrored this back and forth to one another, they learned something about themselves in the other and could then transfer this to their own mothers. The growth of understanding in the group can enable firstly, to take on a mindful sense of responsibility in the moment, and secondly, forgiveness, and then maybe even gratitude to the parents is possible simply for the gift of life. We of course also know from our patients how many of them carry their parents or parts or versions of them for their whole life on their shoulders as a burden, usually in the form of what Freud called the super-ego, the punishing and controlling conscience.

This takes us back to Proverbs and 'the Instruction of thy father' and 'the law of thy mother'. Perhaps these two laws are always in our heads. The law of the father and the law of the mother affect our ways of relating to others throughout our lives. In group analysis, we can assume therefore that various versions of these two laws are always brought into the group by us, as group analysts, and our group members. They are going to be in the group and individual transference, in the group analyst's countertransference and reverie and, above all, in the matrix. Conventionally, the law of the father is the super-ego, the internal voice that says, as in the title of Bernard Barnett's book about the super-ego You ought to! (Barnett, 2007) or what one group patient called 'Musturbation'. Freud said that the super-ego was the heir to the Oedipus Complex, which is of course a set of family relationships, a triangle, in which, in conventional thinking, the father is set up as an interfering policeman. In 1897, Freud said in a letter to Fliess: "the father forbids the child from realising his unconscious wish to sleep with his mother" (Freud in Masson, 1985, p. 75). This is one version of the law of the father and it sometimes appears in the group in the slightly different form of the individual patient, feeling that the group analyst is getting in the way of their relationship with the group, usually by making group analytic remarks and spoiling things for them, as in the group that I mentioned earlier in this chapter.

The view in contemporary psychoanalysis is sometimes rather different and is built into the affirmation of thirdness. This makes more sense in terms of what is known now about the endocrinology of birth and infancy. For example, the father also experiences hormonal changes which affect the brain during the mother's pregnancy and his prolactin levels increase too. This hormone encourages milk production in the mother and stimulates caring behaviour in both mother and father. At the same time, the father's testosterone levels decline, suppressing both aggression and the wish to procreate. The hormonal changes in the father are initiated by the scent of hormone secretions from the mother, which are picked up by the father, and therefore this process is dependent on close physical contact between the parents during the pregnancy. After the birth, both prolactin and oxytocin levels increase, stimulating pleasure and care, but only if the father is lovingly involved with the baby. Happiness and closeness beget more happiness and closeness.

To return to Proverbs again and the law of the mother, Juliet Mitchell (1974) has suggested the concept of the 'law of the mother' as being the mother's prohibition against the toddler killing the new baby. This is a horizontal law, across one generation, whereas the law of the father is vertical, down the generations. Mitchell's assumption is that the aggression, which is forestalled by the 'law of the mother', then turns outwards and the energy feeds into criminality, war and fighting in men, or inwards into melancholia. Again, we are fortunate in group analysis, as every new patient that joins a group is always the hated new baby, and we can never avoid the centrality to all our lives of sibling envy, rivalry and hatred. We also always have to face the drama of thirdness. The group, after all, is made up of triangles, continually alternating with dyads, and that is what gives it its robustness when it is under way. It always happens for us in the present moment, unlike much individual work. The hated and loved baby, sibling and parent are always in the room with us right here, right now, doing what they always do.

Maleness

I want to return, for a moment, to my Y-chromosome. As you know this in humans is what makes me a man, as it contains a gene *SRY*, which triggers male embryonic development. This is only passed on from father to son, from great-grandfather to grandfather to father. The father passes it to his son who gives it to the grandson. Daughters if they have sons will not pass it on, and those male babies will get it from their father.

Because of this exclusively patrilineal transmission process, it is possible to trace the history of the Y-chromosome back to one male ancestor, 'Y-chromosome Adam', who probably lived in East or North-East Africa between 100,000 and 200,000 years ago, when the total population of Homo sapiens humans was less than 16,000 individuals. At the same time, we have an unbroken matrilineal line of decent for our mitochondrial DNA back to 'mitochondrial Eve'. Mitochondrial DNA is passed unmixed from mothers to both male and female children, and all female lineages converge on one individual, also living in East Africa, also between 100,000 and 200,000 years ago. This discovery gave great delight to creationists who imagined that it was scientific proof of the Garden of Eden. They forgot about all the humans before and around them, including Adam and Eve's parents and neighbours, who we are not related to, because sometime in the intervening years, their ancestors did not have either male or female offspring, and whose lineage died out.

This line of thought is interesting, but can be rather confusing, and I have to come back to trying to imagine where I am in the group as a man and a father. Am I being fatherly, paternal, patriarchal or paternalistic? And what is the function or symbolic meaning of each of those in the group at any one moment?

Incidentally, as you can never escape from conscious gendering, which does not always coincide with physical biological reality, and unconscious gendering, which is not in any sense bound by physical and biological reality, where does this come in this debate? Why, for example, do we speak the Mother tongue in the Fatherland? Why do we have Mother Russia and Uncle Sam, Britannia and John Bull? Why are ships female, as in 'all who sail in her'? Why is our parliament the 'Mother of all parliaments'?

Conclusion

These are difficult matters, which we continually come back to. The present difficult and passionate debate about trans-gender is another example of the various forms that this discussion can take. In group analysis, we are fortunate in that the debate is always taking place in front of us in the group, alive in the present moment. What does it mean to be a father or a mother, man or woman, with other men and women, all struggling together to understand? In their unconscious shared life, the group can always be its own father or mother or child, even if only for a moment, in the service of understanding and knowing, and the group analyst can always share, even if only for a moment, as the group-analyst-in-the-group, the search and sometimes what is found.

Chapter 13

The patrix – a new concept for group analysis

Amélie Noack

Introduction

Current models of authority and leadership are often derived from organisational and business management and mainly based on efficiency and profitability. They reflect the more independent and power-related socialisation that men have undergone. Men are traditionally expected to take on leadership roles and their authority is often idealised, while women in leadership positions are more easily denigrated. Research (Rohlfing et al., 2014) has shown that women's socialisation in general supports and favours a more interdependent self-concept. The breakdown of traditional forms of authority and leadership based in male power are becoming visible in the political and economic arenas. I am suggesting that group analytic theory and psychoanalytic thought in general need a fundamental re-balancing in the direction of a co-operation of gendered qualities.

Variety of focus – left and right brain activity

Iain McGilchrist's *The Master and His Emissary* (2009) shows that the Western scientific paradigm has predominately favoured the analytical function of the left brain to the detriment of the more holistic imagery of the right side of the brain. One way to portray the cooperation of the two is the creative process of alternation between focused and diffuse awareness that illustrates the activity of a group conductor, who constantly has to shift focus between the single individual and the group-as-a-whole. The conductor lets things happen on the one hand and allows the group to run itself, and on the other hand may have to grip the reins and conduct events in a focused and controlled way when the going gets rough, since

> The conductor should never have to do the group's work unless and until his help is needed.
>
> (Foulkes, 1991, p. 112)

DOI: 10.4324/9781003310358-18

Giving the permission to focus, then to go off focus and allowing a wider picture, in order to discover another thread and follow it, that is, letting the modes of sharp and wide focus alternate, could be seen as a model for the creative process as such. The alternation between sharp and wide focus has been described as the intercourse between masculine and feminine modes of awareness, but

> today, when masculine and feminine characteristics are so interwoven in people of both sexes, it may be clearer to speak of 'focused consciousness' on the one hand and 'diffuse awareness' on the other, knowing that these qualities belong to both men and women in varying degrees.
> (Claremont de Castillejo, 1974, p. 15)

Leadership and supremacy

Born after World War II, I felt most of my life deep shame about being German and at times haunted by what 'we' had done. An oppressive and authoritarian upbringing intensified this, incorporating relics of traumatic parental war-time experience and the preceding German history suffused by the 'fascist state of mind' (Bollas, 1990). Later, as a foreigner and a German living in Britain, I came across similar attitudes in the socio-cultural matrix here, in that racism and social class were at times denied and hidden behind an egalitarian stance, and so found myself often in the position of a receptacle for shadow projections. For instance, when my first patient group started in 1986 on September 3rd, the first comment from the group was that this was not an auspicious start-date. In response to my question, I was told today was the day that Britain had declared war on Germany in 1939.

In the 1960s, young Germans had begun to confront the terrors of their recent history and challenged the older generation. The abhorrent way in which leadership and authority had been used in the Third Reich informed the anti-authoritarian attitude of the 1960s' students movement. This meant to reject the 'primordial authority of "the father"' (Foulkes, 1991, p. 288), which resulted in an ever increasing gap between the generations. It seemed impossible to imagine positive models of authority and power. By rejecting the authoritarian, fascist need for supremacy, dominance and control, however, my generation was left without any positive model of authority to identify with, but instead had to endure a punitive super-ego and the fear of authority. How would I be able to take on a leadership role in a group on this basis? Would I inevitably have to become an authoritarian father figure?

The challenge of leadership

Discovering and developing authority as a group conductor is a process of blending different qualities. Psychoanalytic theory conveys a clear understanding of the maternal qualities necessary to do analytical work, like the capacity to contain and hold, as it is theorised for example by Bion (1962), Winnicott (1945) and in relation to group work by James (1982a). Paternal qualities are theoretically located in the context of separation, the oedipal struggle and the area of the 'third' (Britton, 1999; Ogden, 1989), but it seems the understanding of the paternal remains somewhat a theoretical abstract. This raised for me the question, if the paternal was implicit within the patriarchal frame of psychoanalytic theory as such. Psychoanalysis is generally taught in reference to Freud, and this is presented as dogma. Considering the paternal as implicit in the patriarchal psychoanalytic frame of reference would explain why observing 'father'-child interaction has not occurred as an area of research – as against mother-infant observation. I believe the results would surprise, especially since father-child interaction can be observed in great detail in every group run along group analytic lines (see Vincent, Chapter 12, this volume).

Is psychoanalytic theory patriarchal?

In this context the difference between the paternal and the patriarchal is important. The paternal describes a particular attitude of relationship, for instance, showing kindness or severity associated with being a father. Patriarchy in contrast describes a system of government controlled by men. Most current-day societies are structured along patriarchal lines, as are most organisations and institutions. Men predominate in politics, hold moral authority in society and control property and social privilege. In psychoanalytic theory, authority may well be resting within the patriarchal body of the theories themselves and be seen as external to the individual practitioner. In contrast, in group analysis, it is expected and in fact required of each practitioner that they use their own personal authority and power when conducting a group. Therefore, a clear understanding of the dynamics of power and leadership are needed as part of group analytic theory, to enable trainees to use authority and power without becoming authoritarian. As Foulkes states in 'Concerning Leadership in Group-Analytic Psychotherapy' (1964)

> the group...shows a need and craving for a leader in the image of an omnipotent, godlike father figure.
>
> (Foulkes, 1964, p. 60)

This regressive need for an all-powerful authority applies to the individual and the group only in the early stages of development, but the inherent glamour and the dangers of this archetypal position has been displayed throughout history by all main leaders. The behaviour of dictators as godlike father figures derives from an identification with the omnipotent masculine God-image inherent in the major monotheistic religions and their particular demonstration of using potency and power. Freud analysed the early human need for the omnipotent father in his last piece of writing *Moses and*

Monotheism (Freud, 1996). He concludes that our relationship to authority is always an ambivalent one. The primitive longing for the primal father's protection on the one hand is always coupled with the adult human need for independence on the other hand. Along with the early human need for the primordial father goes the abdication of personal responsibility and a projection of the redeemer onto the leader. Here lies the basis for totalitarianism, fundamentalism and fascism (Edmundson, 2007). The counterpoint to this is the growing need for freedom in mature adulthood, when challenge, rejection and possibly hatred of godlike authority come into play. Mature adulthood requires from us to take personal responsibility, renounce patriarchal power structures and unmask the illusory allure of omnipotence and omniscience.

A group conductor must, Foulkes (1964) wrote, hold the more primitive archetypal position at the start, when the group needs security and authority. This experience can touch a powerful archetypal level in the group analyst, which can cause inflation and identification with an archetype, which is

> an unconscious identification of the ego's importance to the point of a pathological will to power.
>
> (Jung, 1977, pp. 144–145)

Foulkes was aware of this danger and makes it clear that the conductor holds the archetypal position only in order

> to be able to liquidate it later.
>
> (Foulkes, 1964, p. 59)

since it is the conductor's task that he

> …lets the group, in steps and stages, bring him down to earth. The change is that from a leader **of** the group to a leader **in** the group. The group, in its turn, replaces the leaders authority by that of the group.
>
> (ibid., p. 61)

Embodying the parental couple: matrix and patrix

Every group conductor needs to develop the capacities to be a parental figure – with the very personal blend of their own maternal and paternal qualities – and has to hold the knowledge that this parental position is always only a temporary one, providing a safe space until the group members are able – as a group – to stand on their own feet. While maternal and paternal qualities may be particularly important at different stages of a group's life, the conductor must have access to these qualities throughout the group's life in the form of a combined inner parent or parental couple.

This is a difficult task and explains why it is such a demanding endeavour to run a group competently. In Jungian terms, this would entail the task of bringing the contra-sexual elements of Anima and Animus together in the psyche of the conductor, nothing less than the task of individuation (Jung, 1977).

To support the developing group analyst in this rather arduous task, my proposal from an earlier paper (Noack, 2002b) is reiterated here that it could be fruitful to consider the addition of the term 'patrix' to the group analytic lexicon in order to complement the existing literature about the matrix. The term matrix has been elaborated in a variety of ways (e.g. James, 1982b; Powell, 1989, 1991a; Zinkin, 1998) and describes one of the essential elements of group analysis as fundamentally related to the feminine. MacGregor (2012) reiterated the term 'patrix' in her lecture at the International Group Analytic Summer Conference in Lithuania and also argued that there is a need within group analysis to rehabilitate the father figure.

The term 'patrix' would be the masculine equivalent to the matrix, describing the qualities of benign leadership that are needed by the group conductor. These comprise the basic tasks of dynamic administration together with the maintenance of the boundaries of the group, but also extend to the modelling and 'teaching' of therapeutic behaviour. The importance of teaching and modelling is not stressed enough in the literature, I believe, and is therefore also not sufficiently evident in the training. The therapeutic process of 'translating' an individual's or the group's behaviour (Foulkes, 1964, p. 110f.; 1991, p. 111), like pointing out, clarifying, explaining, linking, confronting or interpreting, are all analytic activities, which the group members will ultimately have to take on as their own task. The ability to perform these tasks is the hallmark of 'ego training in action' (Foulkes, 1990, p. 181), one of the aspects of participation in an analytical group. However, even when the group has matured to take on these tasks, the conductor still

> ...lays down certain conditions, makes the decisions and has the responsibility
>
> (Foulkes, 1990, p. 289)

and

> ...is very active in his own mind...follows the process, ... judges and internally directs all the time.
>
> (ibid., p. 292)

Cooperation: The conductor and the group working together

The group conductor has a parental function in the sense that they create, fashion and instruct the group through interaction with the group. It is this reciprocal interaction which brings the group into being and develops it into a concerted effort, shaped by the group 'and' the conductor. The archetypal background of this combined activity stands in contradiction to the former patriarchal version of leadership in the hands of a single male creator-God, like in Judaism, Christianity or Islam, but must be envisioned, I suggest, in a post-modern way as the function of a creative couple working together as co-creators – matrix and patrix. The idea of a creative couple can be extended to conceptualise the therapeutic work in a group as a co-creation by conductor and group, together, in any given moment. This would develop Stacey's idea that

> [the] matrix as a network...self-organises to produce emergent patterns in its own evolution
>
> (Stacey, 2000, p. 501)

in cooperation with the 'patrix'.

The developing consciousness and awareness of this collaborative process with its capacity to 'draw a line' and to define boundaries relies on the 'patrix', which in Foulkes' words

> ...follows the process, ... judges and internally directs all the time.
>
> (Foulkes, 'The Leader in the Group', 1990, p. 292)

Pines seems to suggest a similar idea of cooperation between maternal and paternal functions in group analysis, when he says:

> When this ongoing group process takes place, then we have both matrix, a basic maternal function, and pattern, a basic paternal function.
>
> (Pines, 1998, p. 98)

With the term 'pattern', Pines refers to Cortesão's contribution to group analysis (David, 2016) in developing the concept of 'pattern', emphasising the conductor's influence through personal characteristics, postures and attitudes. Pattern works like a kind of imprint by the conductor, conveying and sustaining development within the matrix during the group-analytic process. By replacing 'pattern' with the term 'patrix', as I suggest, the conductor's position in the group is highlighted. The conductor's influence is a directive and penetrating activity, fertilising and inserting new impulses into the matrix with the aim of furthering development.

Gerhard Wilke (2014) also argues that it is the work with oedipal material, where mother and father are both objects of awareness, which creates the 'patrix' and makes the matrix strong enough to tolerate a position of 'not-knowing' long enough to allow the known, but not yet thought material to emerge in the group. Authoritarian leadership in the attempt to be the expert and 'knowing it all' forecloses this. It prevents further thinking and any development of better understanding. Keeping an open mind and remaining flexible, personally as well as professionally, is an indispensable quality for modelling benign authority.

Benign leadership of the patrix, where the conductor can tolerate 'not-knowing' what is going on in the group, allows the group itself to find out what is happening. Then

> the group will learn to rely more on itself and be correspondingly more convinced of the truth of its findings.
>
> (Foulkes, 1991, p. 111)

The result of the co-creative endeavour of matrix and patrix – in analogy to the creative act of making babies – moves the therapeutic process on to another level by creating new understanding. A more explicit acknowledgement of the paternal qualities of the conductor's role in combination with the maternal ones and a presentation of these in a clear and thoughtful way during group analytic training is needed. The term 'patrix', denoting firm authority and power used in a benign and thoughtful way combined with the capacity to tolerate creative muddle, confusion and 'not-knowing', could help the conductor to counterbalance the need for control, based in anxiety.

Yet this creates a paradox. It is this paradox which underlies the potency of group work. It is not the personal power or knowledge of the conductor which moves the therapeutic process on, but the power, potency and potential of the group-as-a-whole, including the conductor. The conductor is a member of the group, resonating with the group and using this resonance to further understanding, which more often than not creates "a moment of resonance or unconscious intercommunication" (Foulkes, 1991, p. 119) and so increases the understanding for the group-as-a-whole.

Example

Just before Christmas – the next and last break in the history of the group – Paul declared he had enough. He pronounces defiantly that he will not come back after the break, since the group is going to end at Easter anyway. Paul has challenged my leadership before, without the group taking the issue up. Now a clear response is needed from me to his renewed challenge. I point out that Paul is rebelling and asserting his autonomy like an angry adolescent. Paul responds that he does not like separations and prefers to avoid them, and then adds, rather triumphantly, that he is not willing to talk or think about this any further. I parry this additional attack, saying that he is finally allowing himself to have a tantrum like a three-year-old and is enjoying it fully, imagining that he could destroy us all in his mind by leaving before the end of the group. Now the group joins in. Everybody is trying to help Paul to see how destructive his behaviour is, and people point out that he tends to lose contact and isolate himself when he feels unable to deal with something. The group insists that he needs to change this.

Paul had long longed for a connection with his father. It seemed that this time I found the right tone, since he returns after the break. The group is delighted, someone says: "This must have taken courage".

Paul stayed and worked through the separation process. He ended the group on the last day together with everybody else, saying he had learnt a lot. Experiencing the pain of separation without running away was an important piece of work perhaps not only for him in the group.

Conclusion

The complexity of group analytic processes is difficult to comprehend and to conceptualise. The above example illustrates the effect of cooperation between the working of the patrix – the conductor's use of benign and thoughtful authority and leadership – with the matrix of the group, illustrating the group analytic process of 'ego training in action'.

The infantile human need for omnipotent leadership, which is at the basis of an authoritarian and abusive attitude leading to the patriarchal abuse of power positions, requires a counterbalance in a group analytic theory of benign authority and leadership. For this purpose, it is suggested to add the term 'patrix' to the group analytic dictionary to describe the interactive processes between patrix and matrix, or conductor and group respectively. A group analytical theory of leadership would not only be relevant clinically, but even more so politically, in a world, where totalitarian and fundamentalist tendencies and their inherent dangers are on the rise.

Chapter 14

Normative authority

Sarah Tucker

Introduction

There is a comparatively large literature exploring the nature of the authority of the conductor in an analytic group (e.g. Anthony, 1988; Horne, 1992; Hutchinson, 2009; Nitsun, 2009). This literature generally interrogates the nature of the conductor's authority in the context of the underpinning and essentially democratic frame for group analysis. The flattened hierarchy that goes hand in hand with the democratic frame indicates that the conductor in some way shares authority with the group. Less has been written explicitly about the nature of the authority that lies with the group members and with the group-as-a-whole. In this chapter, I focus on the nature of the authority that resides in the group, introducing the concept of 'normative authority' to capture the quality of it. Before turning directly to this, I outline what I mean by the democratic frame for Group Analysis.

The democratic frame for group analysis

> ...it is in the last resort a political decision or a question of Weltanschauung which [method of leadership] one prefers. One way lies fascism, the other a true democracy.
>
> (Foulkes, 1964b, p. 193)

Foulkes importantly chose the word group 'conductor' to denote the role of the group analyst (Foulkes, 1964a, p. 57). That he did so reflects an essential, hallmark characteristic of the whole group-analytic model, namely, that it is primarily the group that is the authoritative agent of therapeutic change rather than the skill, power or charisma of the group therapist. The flattened hierarchy and democratisation of the locus of authority in groups which is captured by this choice of word was also significant to Foulkes personally, as a refugee who fled from the tyrannical leadership of Hitler's Nazi persecution.

DOI: 10.4324/9781003310358-19

In the context of the democratic frame, the conductor takes a non-directive stance and thus Foulkes says,

> I often felt my contribution similar to that of a conductor. I was not producing; indeed, I refrained from producing the group's ideas, influencing them as little as I could.
>
> (Foulkes, 1975, p. 292)

To honour the democratic spirit, the conductor also needs to be "immune to the temptation to play god" or "act as leader in the usual sense" (Foulkes, 1964a, pp. 54, 64). He conducts the group with both the "courage to lead which springs from his social responsibility" by promoting "co-operation on equal terms between equals" (Foulkes, 1964a, p. 64) so that

> the spirit in which these groups are conducted and the qualities required on the part of the conductor have an essential affinity to education according to the concepts of a democratic way of life for good world citizenship...
>
> (Foulkes, 1964a, p. 64)

This is the democratic frame, where authority lies with and in the group rather than solely with and in the group analyst.

Foulkes describes the role of the leader from two perspectives or levels, the manifest, conscious level of everyday adult contemporary life and the latent unconscious level of historical infantile life (Foulkes, 1964a, p. 57). On the manifest level,

> the group analyst does not assume active leadership of the group
>
> (Foulkes, 1964a, p. 57)

in line with the democratic frame. In sharp contrast, on a latent level, the group

> shows a need and craving for a leader in the image of an omnipotent, godlike father figure
>
> (Foulkes, 1964a, pp. 59–60)

who is also an omniscient and absolute leader with magical powers. In this way, Foulkes suggests that at a latent, unconscious level the group analyst has the position of the primordial leader sketched in Freud's *Group Psychology and the Analysis of the Ego* (Freud, 1921). Foulkes' views about the democratised position of the group analyst as conductor appear to refer largely to his role at the manifest conscious level, while on the latent level, there is a heightened hierarchy in which the group analyst holds considerable power and authority.

According to Foulkes, interaction takes place between the manifest level, where the group analyst is not active in his leadership, and the latent level, where the group analyst is all powerful and omniscience in his leadership. He suggests that, in order to give

> meaning and weight [to] his actions on a manifest level
>
> (Foulkes, 1964, p. 60)

the conductor needs to accept his omnipotent position at a latent level. Here Foulkes points to the way in which the group analyst needs authority at the manifest level to counteract his essentially non-active leadership style and this authority comes from the unconscious transference towards him. This is brought into sharp relief when he talks about

> the ultimate conformity of the group with the...conductor's conscious and unconscious opinions.
>
> (Foulkes, 1971, p. 211)

It is notable that, for Foulkes, the flattened hierarchy and democratisation of the locus of authority in groups is connected with the manifest or conscious life of the group. The democratic frame interacts with but is not itself part of the latent or unconscious life of the group where the group craves an omnipotent leader.

Nitzgen has clearly articulated the importance of the democratic frame for group analysis (Nitzgen, 2001, 2016) as for him, group analysis is, "intertwined with a political impetus" (Nitzgen, 2016, p. 23). He suggests that by locating the power of interpretation with the group members as well as the conductor, Foulkes "stepped out of Freud's shadow and linked Group Analysis indissolubly to democracy" (Nitzgen, 2001, p. 345). Nitzgen highlights one aspect of the democratic flattened hierarchy that characterises the group analytic model, namely the importance and therapeutic agency of group member interventions, such as interpretations, alongside that of the group conductor. He connects this with the democratic frame and brings into relief how this sharply differentiates group analysis from psychoanalysis and points to the political veins of the group analytic model.

Nitzgen argues that according to Foulkes (1964), the group analytic model works for individual members of the group by shifting the culture of the group from one in which there is unconscious transferential love of the 'leader'/conductor as all-powerful at the latent level to a conscious democratic culture in which there is co-operation of equals on equal terms at the manifest level. This transference is dissolved via free-floating discussion leading to ever more articulate communication in the group. Like Hopper (2000), who uses the term 'citizen' to refer to those who have reached a level of emotional maturity, Nitzgen highlights how the democratic culture is considered a mature and healthy one for the individual members in the group analytic model. It is arrived at via the dissolution of their loving transference for the conductor. On these grounds, Nitzgen argues that group analytic training is training in citizenship.

Normative authority and group norms as group-as-a-whole authority

What does it mean to say that, in the context of the democratic frame, authority resides in the group rather than solely with the conductor? I suggest that a fundamental component of this thesis is encapsulated in Foulkes' Basic Law of Group Dynamics (BLGD) which says that,

> the deepest reason why...patients...can reinforce each other's normal reactions and wear down and correct each other's neurotic reactions, is that collectively they constitute the very Norm, from which, individually, they deviate.
>
> (Foulkes, 1948, p. 29)

Individual members of a group will work to weaken and remove support from each other's 'neurotic' or 'abnormal' modes of exchange and will work to strengthen and support each other's 'normal' modes of exchange, which match the norms of the group as a whole, because group members together share these norms.

For Foulkes, a 'neurotic reaction' is a symptom which

> although already a form of communication, ...mumbles to itself secretly hoping to be overheard.
>
> (Foulkes and Anthony, 1957, pp. 259–260)

The language of the symptom is a conscious manifestation of something that the individual wishes to communicate, but the content of which he is as yet unconscious. These symptoms manifest themselves as misfired attempts to relate to other members of the group, in so far as they leave the individual misunderstood and thus isolated in relation to others. The therapeutic work of the group, in the form of free-floating discussion, will serve to translate the misfired communications into a conscious shared language.

According to Foulkes, the BLGD holds that misfired communications of isolated group members do not fit in with the collective group norms. These misfired communications will be weakened, because the group norms are 'collective' and 'permeate' an individual member "all through...to his core" (Foulkes, 1948, p. 30). Being shared at a deep, often unconscious, level, the free-floating group discussion is underpinned by norms for behaviour, which are shared and, according to Foulkes, promote the translation of unconscious misfired communications into a conscious shared group language.

In the operation of the BLGD, we see that the authority, power and rules for behaviour lie primarily in the norms of the group-as-a-whole. These provide implicit guidance and a prescriptive force in the group for how group members ought to communicate and behave. This prescriptive force and authority does not derive from the action of the group conductor in relation to either individual group members or in relation to the whole group, but rather, comes from the action of the normative aspect of the group-as-a-whole.

I suggest that we think of this normative action of the group-as-whole as 'normative authority', highlighting the fact that norms are in and of themselves authoritative. The norms in one group may differ from those in another and so the nature of normative authority differs across group contexts. The concept of normative authority highlights the authoritative nature of group-as-a-whole processes, in contrast to those in association to the maternal matrix. It brings into focus the social and group-as-a-whole nature of authoritative processes at work in groups, by contrast to the individual authority of the group conductor. This reminds us that authority in group analysis is within the democratic frame, and as such lies with and in the group rather than solely with and in the group analyst.

Normative authority and the matrix as group-as-a-whole womb

Normative authority as the operation of normative forces in the group-as-a whole is distinct from the maternal notion of the matrix. The matrix also concerns the group-as-a-whole and is the network of communications and relationships existing between individual members (Foulkes, 1964c, p. 292). It is in this context that 'communication' takes place and it is via 'communication' that the unconscious meaning of neurotic symptoms is translated into conscious communication (Foulkes and Anthony, 1957, p. 129).

Group norms form part of the 'foundation matrix' and so does normative authority. However, it is often highlighted that the term 'matrix' is the Latin for 'womb', a place in which something grows. The matrix is the group-as-a-whole womb, vessel or context in which the unconscious communications in the group are translated into a shared conscious language. The matrix carries for the group-as-a-whole the symbolic role of the mother, providing a safe container for therapy to take place.

This aspect or characterisation of the matrix bears no resemblance to the essential features of normative authority. Firstly, reference to 'the matrix' suggests a reified place or thing that exists within which communication takes place. By contrast, 'normative authority' is intended to capture social 'processes' rather than things. Secondly, the defining features of normative authority – the behaviour shaping and rule giving authority – are, at least traditionally, more associated with the symbolic role of the father in the group-as-a-whole by contrast to the symbolic role of the mother provided by associations to the womb in the concept of the matrix.

The matrix and the patrix

Amelie Noack (Noack, Chapter 13, this volume) notes that by contrast to the symbolic role of the mother with Foulkes' concept of the 'matrix', the symbolic role of the father has been underemphasised in group analytic literature. Noack importantly proposes the introduction of the term 'patrix' to capture a symbolic paternal role in groups. The patrix works alongside that of the symbolic maternal function of the matrix together operating as a 'parental couple'. The patrix denotes,

> The masculine equivalent to the matrix, describing the qualities of benign leadership that are needed... These comprise the basic task of dynamic administration together with the maintenance of the boundaries of the group but also extending to the modelling and 'teaching' of therapeutic behaviour
>
> (Noack, ibid.)

The term 'patrix' is intended to be used specifically to describe a function of the conductor. Thus the 'patrix' refers to authoritative qualities of an *individual*. Normative authority, by contrast, refers to authoritative processes and rules for behaviour as an aspect of the group-as-a-whole. Normative authority refers to social authoritative qualities of the group and in this way is intended to reflect the democratic frame in which authority resides in the group rather than solely with the group analyst.

Normative authority and the superego

Having the capacity for authoritative sway on an individual is a characteristic shared by both the superego and normative authority. However, the two concepts are quite different. Normative authority is conceptually distinct from the psychoanalytic conception of the superego partly because the former is a group-as-a-whole phenomenon while the later resides in the individual. Further, the psychoanalytic superego is a phenomenon concerning individuals, who are not theorised as essentially social, but are understood to have to forge social relationships precisely via the formation of the superego. Freud's account of the development of the superego can be understood to require an inherently antisocial picture of the self, in the sense that the superego allows entry into the social world only via the necessary punitive repression of destructive or unacceptable aggressive and sexual instincts, which are, as it were, unwanted (Freud, 1921, p. 396). The primal aggressive antisocial instinct gratification-driven self needs controlling (primarily by the father), in order to enter into civilisation and deal with the social world. The values of the father are eventually internalised to form the superego.

On this picture, the superego is a secondary response to the aggressive and sexual instinctual aspects of the id to operating in a punitive, authoritarian and behavioural – praise and punishment – manner.

By contrast, in group analysis, Foulkes' essentially social conception of the self is by definition essentially pro-social rather than anti-social. Foulkes does not write explicitly about this view. However, we can turn to Winnicott and see that in his view the cultural social world can be understood to be a result of a primary and creative propensity to relate, articulated in his theory of transitional phenomena (Winnicott, 1953, 1967). A view such as Winnicott's is compatible with the pro-social group analytic model and is in my view implicitly assumed by Foulkes.

An essentially social self has no need to forge a relationship to the social world as the social connections it has are primary, not secondary. On a group analytic social conception for self, where social connections are primary, there is therefore no theoretical requirement for an antisocial and coercive conception of the individual's superego. The Freudian superego is theoretically attached to an instinct driven model of self, which is essentially individualistic and antisocial, giving rise to a punitive and authoritarian authority located in the individual. Normative authority by contrast is theoretically attached to a social model of self, which is essentially prosocial, giving rise to benign authority in the individual's superego, and therefore in the group's-as-a-whole normative authority processes.

Finally, Nitzgen importantly highlights a

> close correspondence between Foulkes' group analytic analysis of the superego and his notion of the Basic Law of Group Dynamics'
>
> (Nitzgen, 2016, p. 27)

Again, the concept of normative authority is different from the group analytic analysis of the superego. It is a group-as-a-whole social phenomenon, while the group analytic analysis of the superego refers to the individual's superego albeit within an essentially social theory of the individual. Normative authority exists over and above the group analytic analysis of the superego, having presumably an essential role to play in its nature.

Example of normative authority at work

Paul, in his forties, never knew his father who died before he was born and is now completely estranged from his mother and his siblings, who his mother always favoured over him. He has a successful professional career and a circle of friends, who he socialises with, but who he does not ever fully confide in. He has had relationships over the years, which have lasted for three to four years, but have all ended with a sense of betrayal for Paul.

By the time he had been in the group for about two years, there had been a number of occasions when, following a challenge from another group member or conflict between him and another group member, he had come back to the next session and announced in his characteristically command-ing professional and accomplished voice that he has considered things care-fully overnight and has decided that he will now leave the group, because he feels there is no place for him in the group. On each occasion, other group members had begun to attempt to open up an exploration with Paul about what had gone on for him emotionally during the previous group session, and on each occasion Paul had remained adamant that he stick to his plan and rejected defensively invitations to explore. At the same time, over the next weeks, the issues dissipated as the life of the group and his place in it moved on and he appeared to forget his plan to leave, as well as the emotional injury.

Over the next year, the length of time Paul could tolerate the exploration of emotions during previous group sessions incrementally increases, so that by the end of his third year in the group, he started feeling safe enough to al-low himself to process his emotional reactions to others with others, rather than solely on his own outside the group. This profoundly opened his capac-ity for intimacy and was accompanied by explorations and interpretations of his behaviour, in terms of his traumatic family experiences of exclusion and betrayal of trust.

In this example, normative authority is at work, slowly and consistently nudging Paul towards his increased capacity to tolerate others in the group sharing his emotional responses. The benign authority does the nudging and the norms include trust and a capacity for dialogue about emotions.

Normative authority, democracy and anti-group processes

With his notion of the anti-group and anti-group processes, Nitsun (1996) challenged Foulkes' democratic thesis that authority in the group lies with and in the group, rather than solely with and in the group analyst. For ex-ample he says that Foulkes' Basic Law of Group Dynamics is 'questionable', because it

> underemphasised the extent to which groups mobilise aggressive and destructive impulses... As such, it did not address the issue of group as opposed to individual pathology.
>
> (Nitsun, 1996, p. 272)

Here Nitsun questions whether the authority of the group as manifested in the BLGD can be trusted, given the possibility of pathological group norms and thus questioning the model of authority in group analysis dictated by what I have described as the democratic frame.

Again, Nitsun suggests that Foulkes' group analytic model is wedded to

an approach to democracy which encourages a spurious sense of equality
(Nitsun, 2009, p. 326)

and cannot deal appropriately with the high level of aggression individuals may bring to the group, which can require strong, active intervention by the group analyst. For Nitsun, there are times in the life of an analytic group, such as when a crisis occurs, when 'aggressive and sexual challenges to authority' and anti-group processes threaten to take hold, "active, not passive, leadership..." is required (Nitsun, 2009, p. 328). For Nitsun, Foulkes'

maximising the authority of the group... does insufficient justice to the power of our relationship with authority.
(Nitsun, 2009, p. 325)

It seems Nitsun appears to reject the authority of the group dictated by the democratic frame in favour of the authority of the individual group conductor.

Normative authority serves to remind us that, whether or not there is aggression in the group or pathology in the group norms, authority and power still resides in the group, be it constructive or destructive. Normative authority thus reminds us that the democratic frame is a given in group analysis. We are reminded that the question of what to do in the face of anti-group processes is not a binary one. It is not about whether the authority should be maximised in the group on the one hand or maximised with the conductor on the other hand. Rather, the question of what to do in the face of anti-group processes is what the nature of the relationship between the conductor and the normative authority of the group-as-a-whole should be in order to withstand social destructive forces.

Indeed Nitsun points towards a picture in which, at the manifest level, there may be a 'wrestling' interaction between the authority of the conductor and the group members (Nitsun, 2009, pp. 340–341), a view which resonates with Horne (1992), who talks about working with the ultimately irresolvable dilemma of control and abdication in group psychotherapy. I suggest that we exchange the 'authority of group members' with the concept of 'normative authority', since this helps to understand that the democratic frame of group analysis is a given. I suggest that in the face of the threat from anti-group processes, we should not give up the democratised locus of authority, in favour of the authority of the group conductor in a binary way.

Conclusion

The concept of normative authority, part and parcel of the democratic frame of group analysis, helps bring into relief the radical and social nature of authoritative processes at work in groups by contrast to the individual authority of the conductor, as well as to the 'maternal' nurturing associations with the group as opposed to the conductor. In the face of anti-group processes, normative authority highlights the need to further articulate how authoritative processes work in the relationship between the group conductor and the normative authority in the group-as-a-whole. Part of this exploration needs to include further understanding of the particular way in which the conductor contributes to the formation of the group norms.

Part 5

Isolation and the social sphere

Introduction

The topic of isolation explores one of the main issues that bring people into therapy. Social isolation, loneliness and feelings of exclusion are on the rise these days, especially since the pandemic caused by Covid-19. But even before, it seemed that more and more people experienced a sense of not feeling part of the society they live in. The beginning of the third millennium has turned out to be a complex and difficult time, individually and collectively, for people and for society, for singular countries as well as globally. Modern developments, globalisation and the rate of rapid change in society require flexibility and mobility rather than support stability and continuity. This increases social isolation, the social isolation of a minority group, the elderly or disabled or of migrants or refugees fleeing a war-torn country. The social isolation that comes with the loss of one's country or the loss of one's family network is even stronger, when there are no other groups for belonging available.

New communication systems have been developed which can make life easier, and the pandemic would not have been manoeuvred as well without these new techniques. The World Wide Web connects us all, but the opportunities come with new responsibilities. Virtual and actual realities need to be differentiated. Communicating with strangers on the internet as if they were friends may undermine intimate and stable attachments through substituting face-to-face relating with online or virtual relating.

The first two chapters look at the role of the internet as a source of connectivity as well as of concealment, and as the possible origin for social and psychic isolation. They point out that group analysis can make an important contribution to the health of individuals and to society as a whole in counterbalancing the effects of psychic and social isolation through offering a space for belonging. Examples are given to illustrate that. In addition, the following chapter explores in more detail the effects of offering experiential groups to students during a training course, pointing to the importance and

DOI: 10.4324/9781003310358-20

positive effects of social connectedness for people, especially when entering a new phase in life, like starting at university.

The final chapter in this part and indeed the book offers an exploration of belonging, inclusion and exclusion by looking at the struggle that belonging entails. This includes a definition of borders and boundaries, friends and enemies. Belonging is a basic human need connected to feeling safe. Fitting in, however, is not always pleasant and being an outsider might be desirable and offer advantages too. Group analysis fosters belonging and offers an experience of it, and our need to belong may well be linked to our anxiety about mortality.

Neil Telfer's chapter was originally presented at a GANLondon Workshop about how internet use affects our lives and impacts on our groups. His group members disclosed that the internet could be a source of connectivity and safety, while compulsively disguising and revealing their emotional vulnerability. The internet, a very influential source of information and connectivity in our culture, can be gratifying, but it comes with emotional costs and its impact is as yet little understood. It is important to hold the creative tension between individual and group in the ongoing struggle towards emotional maturity, insight into oneself and relations with others.

Sylvia Hutchinson's chapter looks at agents of change in group analysis regarding how we group together and relate to one another, especially in relation to social and psychic isolation. This edited version of a talk given in 2015 on the occasion of the 25th anniversary of the founding of the Aarhus Institute of Group Analysis asks if our capacity for reflective thinking and for developing intimate and stable attachments may be undermined by the substitution of online relating for face-to-face relating.

Sandra Evans describes how working with experiential groups as part of a training course differs fundamentally from running therapy groups. Experiential groups are neither therapy nor teaching as such but require the facilitator to combine both pedagogic and therapeutic capacities. They need to engage the students quickly to create a safe space, which reduces anxiety and helps to prevent drop-outs. Working with experiential groups as part of a training course brings benefits not only for the students, who will feel more held and learn to understand themselves better, but also for the organisation they are part of through offering personal connection and engagement.

Sue Einhorn concludes the topic of isolation with an exploration of belonging, inclusion and exclusion by looking at the struggle that belonging entails, a struggle that can feel violent. Being in or out defines borders and boundaries, friends and enemies. When we belong, we feel that we are safe. But being included means fitting in, while being excluded, may mean being scapegoated. Intriguingly, Einhorn links our anxiety about belonging with our mortality.

Chapter 15

Internet and group analysis

Neil Telfer

Introduction

As a Group Analyst, I am interested in how we relate to each other. In my groups, I have experienced how changing patterns of relating are occurring, influenced by internet technology. I hope to show how clinical material brought to light issues of online digitally mediated relating, associated with symptoms, where interpersonal meaning was lost. This challenges group analysis, which is built on communication, relationships and deepening engagement with others and the struggle involved.

Clinical context

In a once-weekly group analytic therapy group, a new member, Tom, had joined for help with his difficulties of feeling stuck in life, isolated, lonely and longing for but afraid of intimate relationships. His background gave a view of his vulnerabilities. His parents separated after a great deal of conflict when he was three years old. His father moved away with his elder brother and Tom stayed with his mother. He felt confused, rejected, abandoned and angry with his parents.

Tom had a history of drug addiction, although not currently, and mood swings of high and low, which left him feeling exhausted. He was now in his thirties, would like a job and to separate from his mother and to have a girlfriend. He introduced himself to the group as an online fantasy 'gamer', who likes to win. He would often stay up all night playing games or watching pornography online, using this to masturbate alone in his room.

In the group, Tom often competed aggressively with others for time and attention. For example, in a session where the group was talking about not being heard or understood by others, a woman asked Tom why he was not participating. Tom responded that he was, "tired and not really interested in her problems" and that the group was not helping him with his problems about separating from his mother and getting a job. The woman said she felt angry about his self-centredness and felt dismissed by him. She then added

DOI: 10.4324/9781003310358-21

that she often felt unable to get through to Tom and connect emotionally. At length, he shouted angrily, "You're all a bunch of losers!" Uproar in the group followed.

I thought this was an example of projective identification of his vulnerabilities as a 'loser' into others. He could not bear the pain or own and articulate his feelings of helpless dependency, instead mapping them onto others.

Tom's use of the internet stood out as extreme. It emerged as a compulsion, escaping into fantasy, online gaming and pornography. The group challenged him. Why was he not going out but avoiding meaningful emotional contact with others in life. He responded that he could not, because he usually got into conflict with others for various reasons. Importantly, he described his online relations with gaming friends as more exciting and easier, and added that face-to-face relations should be as easy.

His remarks elicited empathetic concern and provoked angry reactions from the group – a regular theme. One member noticed that Tom was pushing others away, said he felt rejected and dismissed. He questioned Tom: "Well, why are you here in the group?" Tom didn't respond. Another member said he needed to grow up and get real. Tom's wish to control others was felt and expressed by the group. He was regarded as a 'know all' and would not listen. I thought that he was resisting looking at himself. Also, as in all symptoms, his behaviour hides problems and reveals something important. I thought he was revealing his anxiety and defences, in getting things back to front in that he wanted ordinary real relating to be like virtual relating. He was in fact lonely, and not developing as he would like in life despite all his connections with online 'friends'.

The group discussed the differences between internet use in daily life for information, contact with friends and even pornography, but also acknowledged the need for having some sort of boundary between real and virtual life. They also talked about what is desired, as we all have fantasies and the painful awareness of what is available and what is not. Tom did not participate. He further distanced himself from others in the group when he said pointedly that he had come for help and would like his problems (isolation, loneliness) solved. He simply wanted to be given an answer. The group responded by saying he was new, would need to be there for longer, join in the struggle to get to know others and himself by engaging in conversation, and not be so demanding and controlling.

Although this is a complex dynamic field, I believe this exchange highlighted his group problem. He shows he has difficulties relating to others satisfactorily, pushing them away. He denies his neediness, hates his feelings of helpless dependency and terror as though showing others his vulnerability by opening up would be risking further unbearable rejection. This was taking place in a group where others were also struggling to face their own vulnerabilities. Tom often remained in a concrete state of mind and removing himself from emotional contact. He would often say "I need you to be more concrete", "Tell me what to do", "How do I do that?" A common response by the group was that, although painful, it takes a while to get to know others and them you.

Symptoms to transference

Although there were many other issues emerging in the complexity of the group, a recurrent theme was of frustrated interactions with Tom about his frequent attempts to evade emotional contact with others. I thought he was stuck, unconsciously trying to make the group familiar, like his family in the transference, where he was the child to be looked after and not to grow up emotionally. My countertransference was of feeling frustration and deep sadness. The more he avoided his feelings, the stronger these feelings became in the group, who had to hold them for him. In this, he was recreating his isolation too. An important element of this was his emerging terror of rejection and abandonment in the present, especially at endings of sessions and holiday breaks, which linked to his past trauma, the break-up of his family when very young and when he felt rejected, abandoned and very angry. Tom had real difficulties with boundaries. Although not alone in this, he exhibited an increased anxiety towards the end of sessions about separation and having to wait a week for the next group. He proposed a solution, suggesting the group meet up outside group times. He had no friends and wanted to make friends with other group members. He also asked a woman out on a date, which was declined firmly with the woman adding that she felt unsafe. She was here for therapy not to date!

One member, in an empathic way acknowledging his anxiety, asked him to come out in the group and play, like ordinary people, as separation was something that affected all of the group. He responded that he had been afraid to go out to play with other children when younger and that he could never be ordinary. The group challenged him on this. Why not? He said in what I experienced as a distancing, grandiose tone "Because ordinary rules do not apply to me". The group commented on the irony with dismay that he plays online yet would not play with them in the group. Clearly, they wanted him to join in, build a relationship, get to know him, so he could learn and grow. His need for control out of anxiety was a defence against depression – the result of traumatic loss, rejection and abandonment as an infant.

The group questioned his use of the internet, especially with gaming and pornography as it affected his attendance at the group. They pointed to the attention and importance he was paying to online 'relating' but being unavailable in the group itself. A pattern emerged following 'difficult' group sessions. An increase in his gaming or pornography use online, sometimes all night long, led to him being late for the group, arriving in an exhausted state or not attending the group at all. The group confronted him for 'hiding' on the internet, a substitute for not going out and avoiding contact with others.

He denied this and said at first, it's only a game, then, that he had an addiction to the internet, as if he had no control over his behaviour. However, the internet enhances what is already there within the subject, illustrating according to Wood (2007, p. 164) the psychic reasons for the behaviour.

In another session, he sexualised his relationships in the group, as he told a woman that he would "like to cum on her face". She was shocked and angry, asking him why he wanted to humiliate her? He could not answer and seemed surprised by her response. He had acted on impulse, not thought about it or the context, but when pressed by others to say how he felt, he said he was angry with her, because he felt he could not get into the group discussion other than to say what he was thinking. The group linked his hostile erotic way of expressing himself and the consequences of this in 'real' relating to his online porn fantasy. This interaction proved useful, because his behaviour was immediately responded to in the present by real others. He apologised, which acknowledged his relationship with the woman and acting destructively with anger.

I think this episode also revealed an unconscious scenario, giving meaning to his obsession with online pornography, here emerging as acting out. I thought he was, as posited by Turkle (2011), defensively blurring the distinction between virtual and real face-to-face relating in the transference while rejecting others in the group. Moreover, I suggest this dynamic shows that he took a 'superior, vengeful, triumphant' position, where

> the 'other' is seen to suffer and their suffering is a source of satisfaction and pleasure. In this defensive reversal the original 'victim' becomes the victor. Trauma becomes triumph and passive suffering becomes active revenge.
>
> (Wood, 2007, p. 173)

Online he was free to project his fantasies onto others. There was no real relationship or immediate feedback to learn from.

Some progress was made in a shift during one heated exchange in the group, when he told us that he pretended he didn't feel anything, because if he did he would feel so depressed. The group showed empathy at his honesty and made it clear they preferred him to be more real than false. This showed too that he had the capacity to think and relate if he wanted to. The group reminded him of this when he was blocking them and asked him to take responsibility for himself and limit his passive aggressive way of relating.

I believe too that as a 'winner' in online gaming, others are needed to carry loss for Tom, so that the distress of his primary loss can be evaded. He tried to do this in the group, but was confronted, questioned and challenged at a time, when he could reverse his projections and begin to get in touch with the reality of his losses and started mourning while engaging with others. At times, he did so by weeping, establishing a more authentic connection with himself and others. This dynamic provided lots of material to think about in the therapeutic space, which then could act as a mirror to see ourselves and to reflect on as individuals in relation to others, creating greater cohesion and coherence.

Discussion

Tom's way of relating was often foregrounded in the group, particularly his difficulties with separation and boundaries. This reminded me of an infant's desire for constant presence and struggle to separate, a feature of failed dependency needs, often associated with addictive behaviour. He still lived with his mother but wanted to move away. By defending against relating in the group, he was resisting internalising relationships which could help him grow emotionally.

The meaning of group breaks and separations is a challenge and achievement for all and an important part of treatment. Freud in his 1917 paper *Mourning and Melancholia* (Freud, 1917) describes that the internalisation of the relationship with the lost object concludes healthy mourning. This illustrates Tom's problem with separation. He needed the group to be present and was very anxious about being alone. Yet when he could accept trusting and belonging to the group, he could continue this important mourning process. Trusting, belonging, listening and taking in relationships with others meant he was separate. The appeal of online relating for Tom was, I believe, that others are not experienced as separate, but as part objects to project his needs into whenever and however he wishes. Separations, breaks and losses occur all the time, but if rejected and abandoned too early in life, a break can feel like an actual abandonment and terror of annihilation. However, if enough psychological work has been done, a connection remains. I point out to the group that we are having a break – and will start back on a future date.

I believe that Tom's isolation was very sad. If thought about as a symptom, it can reveal a lot. He was in fact lonely, despite all his connections with online 'friends'.

The task of the therapeutic group in group analysis is translating such an isolating symptom into shared conversation in the group. A basic principle of group analysis is that the origin of dis-ease lies between people. Neurosis is individualistic and destructive to the group, because an aspect of the self is isolated and cannot be expressed in words within relationships. Its origin points to an incompatibility between the individual and their original family group. Thus, symptoms need to be translated and shared through language, which makes communication a central concept in group analysis (Behr and Hearst, 2005, p. 11).

What struck me most was that Tom's online compulsion was being used as an alternatively easier and more desired way to relate while it exploited his vulnerabilities. His unmet needs became an organising principle for relating with others, while unconsciously blocking engagement with others in the group and preferring online to face-to-face relating, he made the aggressive, sexually explicit remark to the woman group member. The group linked this experience to his fantasy pornography compulsion, but now, in person in the presence of the other, it had real consequences, which was analysable in distinguishing fantasy and reality. I believe, he was genuinely shocked and consequently better able to discriminate between the two.

The internet supplied objects which were attractive to him. Given his background and presenting problems, the contrast between vulnerability in the group and power on the internet was salient. His use of the internet as a means, or mediator, in relating to others through games and pornography respectively, were always on his terms. I understood this as a 'psychic retreat' according to Steiner (1993), which are states of mind into which patients withdraw to evade anxiety and mental pain, but this inevitably leads to getting stuck and restricted in life generally. More fundamentally, in terms of classical psychoanalysis symptoms are behaviours caused by the return of repressed psychic material. Insistent desires that the individual feels they must repress will often find alternative paths toward satisfaction and therefore manifest as symptoms. A symptom according to Freud (1926) is a sign of and substitute for an instinctual satisfaction which has remained in abeyance and is a consequence of the process of repression (Freud, 1926, 20.91). Symptoms tend to be activities that are detrimental to one's life; in extreme cases, such symptoms

> can result in an extraordinary impoverishment of the subject in regard to the mental energy available to him and so in paralysing him for all the important tasks of life.
>
> (Freud, 1926, p. 35)

I suggest Tom was unconsciously creating a psychic retreat on the internet. This was not just a compulsion and reinforcement of his defences against his core pain of dependence by omnipotence and manic highs, in which the boundary between online and face-to-face relating became distorted and the subject-object distinction became blurred. I saw this hypothesis supported by unconscious confirmation in his characteristic object relating and responses to it. Online Tom could maintain omnipotent control. Online is like being in

> space, the person is weightless, free from the constraints of relationships and the vulnerability bestowed by our ties and our limitations...
>
> (Wood, 2007, p. 163)

The internet is indeed a technological advance with enormous scope and power. From a psychoanalytic point of view, those very qualities of the internet, which render it powerful, also bestow a potential for manic excitement and omnipotence. With the smallest gesture, the click of the mouse, the individual can control what happens, the part that they wish to play and decide exactly when it should end. The individual can pursue sexual fantasies without any reliance on another person. In the use of pornography, there is no unpredictable other, who might accept or reject, cherish or criticise. With both pornography and chat rooms, the person can avoid the exposure entailed in intimacy with a partner, that is, exposure of the physical body and aspects of themselves they feel ashamed of or vulnerable (Wood, 2007).

> The internet has the power to turbo charge, that is, to accelerate and intensify online sexual activity. Internet pornography is said to be the crack cocaine of pornography.
>
> (Wood, 2007, p. 163)

The nature of Tom's retreat to the internet functioned not just as pastime or diversion with pleasures but had consequences. It became a symptom and entailed hiding self-knowledge which did not need to be faced. In Tom's case, I believe, it served his need to counter feelings of helpless dependency with triumph, like a manic high (Wood, 2007).

In her book *Alone Together*, Sherry Turkle (2011) suggests internet technology becomes like a psychological symptom, obscuring a problem by 'solving it', but without addressing the deeper meaning. Crucially, when technology functions like a symptom, it disconnects us from our real struggles (Turkle, 2011, p. 283).

I suggest that Tom's dilemma was his compulsion to virtual, online 'relating'. This demands immersion in simulation, leading to further simulation (Turkle, 2011) without seeing the limitations or differences between what he needed and what he thought he needed. It left him depleted and fearful of real relationships.

The internet as a way to learn about relating?

I worked on developing my ideas on distinguishing between online and face-to-face relating in preparation for helping the group with this struggle.

> Group analysis is concerned with the **total** behaviour of the individual and we wish him to become himself aware of its meaning and to change his behaviour when it leads him to difficulties.
>
> (Foulkes, 1971, p. 209)

I consider this a call for the group analyst to pay attention to signs of unconscious material, not just what is said, but including deeper communication. Communication via digitally mediated relationships (DMR) occurs on a surface level. Although useful, this can be problematic. There are overlaps and divergences between both systems, and I wanted to discover how dialogue can break down by exploring some of the relevant organising principles of internet use and group analysis respectively, without splitting them into good or bad. My aim is to stimulate thinking and discussion without polarising the issues.

Turkle (2011) argues that we now expect more from machines than from each other. Using the internet changes the way we see ourselves and others, blurring the distinction between self and object. As a result, we need to analyse surface levels of digital communication, many of which converge or diverge, complement and contradict, to learn how accurately surface reflects depth meaning, the signified.

> When technology is a symptom, it disconnects us from our real struggles.
> (Turkle, 2011, p. 283)

I linked this to Tom, who I believe, used the internet defensively to express and hide his symptoms.

> We love our objects, but enchantment comes at a price.
> (Turkle, 2011, p. 283)

He regularly assumed others were like him without questioning his assumptions or validating them in dialogue with others. The group often challenged his attitude and linked it to his fantasy gaming and pornography as contrasted with real, in-person relating.

On the internet, with digitally mediated relating, mutual understanding and agreement can be difficult to achieve and this can lead to conflict. Without an immediate real response from others, how can we understand the meaning created and the processes used to communicate? How do we learn to differentiate between what is included or excluded, suppressed and unstated when we communicate? This would work best if there were an awareness and shared understanding of the meaning created. But in actuality things may not be like that and may either be taken for granted or hidden or both. In 'space', the person is weightless, 'free from the constraints of relationships and the vulnerability bestowed by our ties and our limitations' (Wood, 2007).

Group analysis as social mediator

Group analysis could be understood as a mediator of social modes of relating which could illuminate the difficulties of my patients. Joining a group analytic group helped Tom to deepen his way of relating to others in a more meaningful way without which he could not make relationships, essential for his emotional growth. I also believe this, in turn, helped the group to understand something about building meaningful relationships. In other words, making the unconscious conscious, stating the unstated, the important need for boundaries involved in the different contexts of face-to-face and virtual relating become explicit.

Exploring communication and the need for boundaries leading to real freedom is grist to the mill in group analysis. For instance, Tom would contact me outside of sessions, when he felt the space between sessions or separation to be unbearable. Other patients also send text messages to me at some time. This kind of behaviour can be understood as undermining the relationship between the patient and the group, unless it is addressed by bringing the communication back into the group.

I believe what I have described is an example of a wider cultural expectation, in that the availability of the internet has made us believe that we can have whatever we want at any time. This expectation, however, undermines the value of attachments and separations and the ability to develop more realistic and firmer boundaries of self and other and the attempt to build sustaining relationships.

Getting to know each other, deepening rapport, communicating and relating is vital in group analysis. The link between identity and the sense of belonging to a group underlines the importance of the social field and the role of others in our development. Group analysis is founded on the premise that people are social beings. When things go wrong, we turn to others for help. Turning to a machine for a technical solution can be useful, as Turkle (2011) argues, but can also be problematic, when addressing human needs – a more precious thing.

The importance of meaning and belonging

The dynamics in my group helped me to compare and contrast DMR with an optimum group analytic process. Members join and at first feel isolated and preoccupied with 'their problem' until they learn to belong to a matrix or network of relationships. When that has happened they can be more open to listening, relating, communicating and connecting with others. This is often the real problem, although it could not be articulated by the individual member until helped by the group's responses to them (Garland, 1982).

This process is difficult to grasp and has to be experienced as an interplay between subject and object, which allows a de-centring of the self as the group matrix is taken on board by each individual in the group. Van der Kleij (1985) elaborates the idea that de-centring is the difference between what goes on in our minds and what we experience around us. In the presence of a group we have to deal with the common experience of feeling de-centred, being penetrated by mental processes around us.

It is as if the members of the group are words in a sentence, none of whom can express their meaning except as objects – unless they belong to each other. We need to belong to be able to express and deal with the difference between what we experience and what else is going on in our minds. If we remain de-centred, or isolated from each other, we can only be in our problems, deprived of their meaning because we are disconnected from the total syntheses, which we need to survive.

(Van der Kleij, 1985, p. 107)

I suggest, that if we are to grow and understand ourselves and our relations with others, body to body, shared meaning is needed rather than information. Meaning is created by being shared in a common context, through the experience of being with others. Ideally, this process involves both a de-centring 'and' an integration of identity, belonging to the group with a greater chance of understanding something together. However, like all techniques, group analysis has limitations too. The problem is believing that technology can solve everything. "All creativity has a cost" (Turkle, 2011, p. 283).

Conclusion

It can be difficult to grasp how internet technology affects us, although it is clear that we are shaped by it in ways we need to understand. This insight emerged as my group struggled to engage with each other and build communication links and relationships.

In this chapter, I sought to examine deeper organising principles of internet and group analytic functioning to help understand how mediation can work in either domain. In cyberspace, digitally mediated relationships extend us in a kind of disembodied consciousness, where the meanings created are not our own. This is both seductive and has consequences, making us feel anxious about our personal boundaries. In extreme cases, with vulnerable people, I have found, it can blur the distinction between self and other as Turkle (2011) posits, and then functions like a symptom.

I suggest that if we only see the internet as an alternative and easier way of 'connecting' to others, but fail to see the limitations and the values, implicit in its use as a virtual mode of relating and needing to be contextualised, this can lead to a loss of meaning in building the sustaining, ordinary social relationships we all need to develop and grow.

Chapter 16

Psychic and social isolation

Sylvia Hutchinson

As a group analyst in the later stages of my career, I have been preoccupied by how our changing world is impacting on the practice of psychotherapy, and on group analysis in particular. Globalisation and accelerated technological, environmental and social change have brought profound changes in the way that we group together, and the way we communicate and relate with one another. My impression, based on my experience both inside and outside the clinical field, is of an increase in social and what I have called 'psychic' isolation that is taking place, despite the extraordinary and invaluable opportunities to 'connect' that modern technology has brought. It is my view that this increased 'connectedness', though it might help introduce people to one another and keep people connected, does not necessarily protect and foster the capacity to establish and maintain stable attachments and intimate relationships in the way that, I think, group analytic groups might do.

Foulkes, writing with James Anthony (Foulkes and Anthony, 1957), had this to say already fifty or sixty years ago:

> The first and foremost aspect with which group psychotherapists are usually concerned and according to which they form their concepts, is that of belonging, of participation. Being a respected and effective member of the group, being accepted, being able to share, to participate, belong to the basic constructive experiences in human life. *No health is conceivable without this.* [my italics]
>
> (Foulkes and Anthony, 1957, p. 27)

And this:

> The relative isolation, alienation, of the individual is thus a very real problem of our time.
>
> (Foulkes and Anthony, 1957, p. 24)

Along with group analysts such as Morris Nitsun (2014) and Elizabeth Rohr (2014), who have written of their concerns about the challenges facing us

DOI: 10.4324/9781003310358-22

as group analysts in our dramatically changing world, I too would like to see group analysis extend beyond the clinical and organisational fields – to be on offer as a psychosocial intervention to counter the invisible forces that may be undermining our capacities for intimate relating. Group analytic groups, aimed at promoting self-awareness and understanding, could provide communities with some protection from the possible undermining effects of forms of communication that can encourage the 'objectification' of the individual and the humanising of machines. This speaks to my ever-growing belief in the power of group analysis to transform, repair and provide healing and corrective group experience. I do not think that this is an idealisation of group analysis as I am well aware of its limitations – and of the difficulties, pitfalls and risks associated with setting up and maintaining group analytic groups.

My first experience of personal therapy was in a group analytic group run by Robin Skynner in the early seventies. Having emigrated from South Africa to the UK a few years previously, this group analytic group offered me more than a 'corrective experience' of dysfunctional family dynamics – it also offered opportunities for integration into English society and offered structures that, in the absence of any available family, social and other groups of belonging, protected against the deleterious effects of isolation on both mind and body.

Social isolation may be structured into our lives by circumstances, where we happen to be in a time and a place and social position, whether it be the social isolation of a migrant or of a refugee, fleeing a war-torn country to seek safety in an unfamiliar culture, where there are no available groups of belonging, or the social isolation that comes with the loss of the integrity of the family or the extended family network. Our particular social circumstances and context will play a significant part in whether or not we find ourselves in positions of relative social isolation.

Elisabeth Rohr, in her 2014 Foulkes lecture (Rohr, 2014), has suggested that modern developments, globalisation and the accelerated rate of change in our structures and institutions – developments that favour mobility and flexibility rather than continuity and stability – undermine the human capacity to bond and experience intimacy. A loss of such capacity can only increase what I have called psychic isolation, and by this, I mean 'being *emotionally* cut off within one's relational network'. Here, unlike the experience of isolation through social circumstances that may be age-related or to do with social exclusion through being a member of a minority groups, the disabled, the foreigner, etc., psychic structures that have emerged to survive developmental trauma and deprivation may be further weakened by the loss of continuity and stability in our relational worlds.

Bringing people out of isolation, being part of a network and the experience of belonging, that can accompany being part of a resonating matrix, are therapeutic factors that have taken on a greater urgency in the search for emotional and physical health and well-being. Nearly seventy years after the publication of Foulkes's *Introduction to Group-Analytic Psychotherapy* in 1948, we live in a different world today. Every aspect of our lives is now being shaped by digital technology. There is a growing awareness of a future that is difficult to predict. We see both creative and destructive processes transferred to cyberspace, like internet activism, bullying on the internet, fraud (identity) and theft. And the implications for psychotherapy practice are currently being debated – around clinical issues, ethical issues, online and teletherapy, the use of Zoom and so on.

What we know is that the balance between face-to-face and machine-mediated communication is changing and tipping increasingly towards machine-mediated communication. Our access to each other and to information is now held at our finger-tips on our mobile phone in the palm of our hand, allowing us twenty four hours connectivity. And we can disconnect at the flick of a finger! We are nodes in an incredibly complex, worldwide network.

Our new technologies erode existing boundaries in many *different* respects: (i) the boundary between man and machine; (ii) time and space boundaries collapse; (iii) between work and leisure; (iv) between private and public; (v) between phantasy and reality; (vi) between representation of reality, the virtual and reality; and (vii), most significantly, between self and other. These boundaries dissolve and reform in new and different configurations. New rules govern our patterns of attachment and separation, of intimacy and social relating. Online groupings for instance establish their own norms, codes of conduct and cultures.

Sherry Turkle, a psychoanalytically trained psychologist and professor and director of the MIT Initiative on Technology and the Self, expressed the view in a recent TED talk (Turkle, 2013), that the increased use of machine-mediated communication is undermining our capacity for solitude, for listening to each other and for self-reflection. She suggested that we are sacrificing conversation for mere connection and that with the ease of remaining connected twenty-four hours a day we live with the illusion of never having to be alone.

Winnicott (1958) in his paper 'The Capacity to be Alone' considered this one of the most important signs of maturity in emotional development. He links the capacity to be alone to having the experience of 'good-enough mothering' and thus building a belief in a benign environment, rather than the expectations of a persecutory one. To quote Winnicott:

> the ability to be truly alone has as its basis being alone in the presence of someone.
>
> (Winnicott, 1958, p. 33)

This is usually mother.

In this way an infant with weak ego organisation may be alone because of reliable ego-support... and gradually the ego-supportive environment is introjected.

(Winnicott, 1958, pp. 33–36)

And he concludes that

without a sufficiency of this experience the capacity to be alone cannot develop.

(Winnicott, 1958, pp. 33–36)

It is my view that the creation and maintenance of a group analytic situation and a group analytic attitude offers ideal conditions to provide compensatory experiences to build on this capacity – either for those who have been deprived of good-enough mothering (many of whom we see in our clinics) or for future generations hooked more exclusively into connectivity rather than relationship. The group analytic group as 'environment mother', that is as a dynamic matrix with the presence of an inhouse therapist, can in principle provide this reliable, stable and safe enough secure base to enable venturing out, experimenting and trying out new ways, potentially consolidating the capacity to be alone. Turkle (2011) has described our increasing addiction to 'being connected' as more like a symptom than a cure. Here is an example of translating such a 'symptom' in a group analytic therapy group.

Example

A member of a weekly therapy group regularly sat in the group with her mobile on her lap, the sound was off but she would be constantly attending to it. Following some rather half-hearted attempts to challenge her, she was confronted rather more forcefully by an older member. She then disclosed that she kept her mobile on at all times, since she was addicted to it and couldn't bear the thought of a missed communication. Much to the group's surprise another group member, considered the more mature father-figure in the group, owned up to keeping his phone on vibrate throughout the group and that he too would have difficulties switching it off. There followed a discussion in the group about relationships to mobiles and about twenty-four-hour communication access. We looked at our young members' dependency relationships and linked her mobile addiction to her early history of intense separation anxieties, which was the major issue with which she entered the group. Early on she reported having to phone her mother every day, both to keep her mother alive and to allay her anxieties about loss. In an intimate and highly charged atmosphere, the group then moved to sharing anxieties about dependency and experiences of failed dependency. Since then she no longer keeps her mobile on her lap.

In this example, the mobile phone appears to function as a self-object, what Kohut and Wolf (1978) described as an early object (or person) that functions to regulate the emotional state. The group members' separation anxiety transferred to an anxiety about losing connection with her phone. Keeping her phone at hand and switched on helped regulate her anxiety, both about being in the group, and about being separated from mother.

In our group analytic groups, where we engage in multiple relationships and try to make sense of them, misunderstandings can be corrected and shared meaning found. The emphasis on feeling, thinking and reflection may also provide an antidote to the possible undermining effects of increased machine-mediated communication, and thus both protect and facilitate the development of our reflective capacities.

I have wondered whether the rising popularity of mentalisation-based therapies (Bateman and Fonagey, 2006) and the seeming increase in the diagnosis of borderline personality disorder (BPD) is in part a reaction to a threat to reflective thinking arising from changing patterns of communication. Bateman and Fonagey (2006) also highlight two pre-reflective modes of thought that antedate mentalising or meaning making: (i) the 'psychic equivalence' mode, where you believe I think like you think, and where there are difficulties separating my mental state from your mental state, and (ii) the 'pretend mode', which is a detachment from reality. The virtual world provides infinite arenas for play and experimentation, for self-construction, for joining groups and forums, without the reality testing and constraints of face-to-face relationships. The time spent between disembodied and embodied relating is shifting, increasingly towards disembodied relating.

We now can present ourselves as we want to be and can control and regulate the distance between self and other. This creates what Sherry Turkle (2013) calls the 'Goldilocks effect' – the three bears were not there to give feedback! I anticipate that with increasing use of the internet to communicate with others, we may see new syndromes developing that are characterised by excessive reliance on 'pretend mode', the absence of reality testing and perhaps also resorting to psychic equivalence mode. I believe that group analysis has a major contribution to make to the health of our society as a whole, as well as for those whose lives have been derailed.

Concluding remarks

I would like to conclude with another snapshot from a therapy group. The experience of belonging and being part of a network is an ongoing process, but there are moments, often moments of resonance in the group, when this is amplified – and highlighted:

A patient, Sarah, joins the group, and within a few months develops a pattern of irregular attendance, often for work reasons, sometimes for other reasons. Some members of the group experience this as an attack and a devaluing of the group – and confront her. Sarah tells the group that she does not feel better after groups and that she is not sure this is doing her any good. The moment when the group linked her flight from the group with her flight from her family, when, as a child and adolescent she spent as much time outside the family home as possible in order to escape from 'being made to feel bad', was an epiphany moment for her – and a point of shared meaning for the group. It was at this point that it felt like she joined the group and became part of it – and group members were more able to understand and contain her.

Catching a re-enactment, like this, live, in the here and now, is often a significant moment in becoming connected and feeling part of the group – a moment where we can see someone coming out of isolation.

Chapter 17

Teaching and learning in small groups – maximising learning and minimising anxiety in an experiential group

Sandra Evans

Introduction – the small experiential group

This chapter is based on the experience of teaching on an MSc course on the 'Theory and Practice of Psychological Therapies' and sets out the relevant details by using the theoretical framework of learning in groups.

As a group analyst providing experiential groups in a teaching setting, I realised that there exists a tension between the Foulksian non-interventionist approach of medium- and long-term group analytic psychotherapy and a need for more structure in order to engage students over the short period of a teaching term lasting only three months. The group analytic approach as such lends itself well to teaching students about the power of groups through being in a small experiential group, which is an appropriate medium both for therapy and teaching. It offers the opportunity for an exploration of the unconscious, provides mutual support, and fosters self-awareness and personal growth. Interactions between members are both creative and unpredictable, which makes for exciting work, even if a little daunting at times. There is also potential for darker moments in the group (Nitsun, 1996), like scapegoating, so the facilitator's knowledge of group dynamics and how to harness them is helpful.

Clinical skills teaching for medical undergraduates and psychiatry trainees, particularly involving simulation techniques, use the principles of experiential learning (Kolb, 1984) and are structured in a way that lends them well to techniques encouraging interaction in small groups (Light and Cox, 2009). The students are not required to be in personal therapy, as the course is explicitly a theoretical programme and does not qualify to see patients. However, for teaching quality purposes and as an innovation, the students are offered an experiential group, a group which is neither didactic nor structured, nor is it psychotherapy. The experiential group offers a reflective space (Schon, 1987), in which to experience and appreciate some of the theoretical knowledge taught in more traditional ways in lectures, seminars, etc. and can have a beneficial effect on students. To encourage that,

DOI: 10.4324/9781003310358-23

the facilitator invites the group at the start to explore unconscious processes (Freud, 1915) through what happens within the boundaries of the group.

Development of the course – learning by doing

The experiential groups of the MSc in Psychological Therapies have grown in size since the course's inception. After a few years, three additional group analysts were engaged to facilitate the groups. With more than forty students enrolled and with ten as an optimal number of members for these groups, more staff were needed. Having colleagues to discuss the groups in a somewhat supervisory fashion also offered a greater opportunity to reflect on process. Together we noted problems in the groups that were possibly a reflection of the learning environment, but were also, to some extent, mirroring the struggles of the students themselves. These issues presented opportunities to learn, develop the module and improve the learning experience for the students.

We synthesised group processes and dynamics with pedagogic theory in order to bring a different understanding of the nature of experiential learning. In the conclusion, some of these thoughts are summarised in order to optimise the conditions in which to engage students and help them reach a deeper understanding of the psychological. Throughout the text, some constructive thoughts and suggestions are emphasised in order to improve planning for future groups.

Learning through experience

On the course, the experiential group is presented in direct comparison to two other methods of small group teaching, which are commonly run in medical schools: a problem-based learning (PBL) module and a communication skills session using simulated patients.

One essential issue is the tension between 'having an experience' versus the need to engage students, initially at least, with theory and a rationale. Being immersed in feeling and experiencing at 'firsthand' what is described in the literature can be anxiety provoking. Without sufficient theoretical structure, there may be a danger of inducing overwhelming anxiety (Bion, 1961), which may prevent the students from engaging or turning up at all. The Foulksian experiential group is indeed an intense version of small group teaching used across the undergraduate medical curriculum. However, it is a very powerful learning tool and the literature suggests that experiential learning is effective and provides a form of 'deep learning' (Biggs, 1987). There are however problems inherent in it that may exclude some learners, particularly those who find self-reflection problematic. It is important to be aware of this and minimise the fallout, while maximising and enhancing the learning experience. In experiential group teaching, students need to be engaged early on. Without the usual structure, their curiosity needs to be stimulated to stick with the programme.

Reflections and suggestions for future planning

In these groups of would-be psychologists and clinicians, their curiosity is likely to be stimulated by altruistic feelings towards their patients. The group offers some degree of authenticity in that respect, because listening to other members will help understand the lived experiences of patients and constitutes an opportunity for getting in touch with one's own and others' unconscious processes. Providing a prior teaching session, like describing the therapeutic factors in groups (Yalom, 1985) along with Bion's 'Experiences in Groups' (1962), is enough to provide the basic framework in which to engage students. Making group attendance mandatory and communicating this clearly is also helpful.

Structure of the experiential groups

In terms of demographics, the majority of postgraduate students taking this master's degree are women with degrees in psychology, nursing, medicine or allied professions. Sixty percent are from overseas with about twenty percent from non-European countries. The experiential group is offered in the second term of three in the full-time course. The group described here ran as a programme of five fortnightly sessions of ninety minutes. The challenge for the facilitators was to give the students a positive experience of being in a group, while learning in a very short time about the unconscious (Freud, 1915) and 'whole group' processes (Foulkes and Anthony, 1984). In this course, the relevant theory teaching, a single lecture on group dynamics, followed at the end of the module. Prior to the group starting, students had been taught psychodynamic theory, but had not had any specific group related information.

Reflections and suggestions for future planning

From the applied learning perspective it is generally more helpful to have the theory lecture first, rather than at the end, but this also risks the potential for diluting the actual experience by making students anticipate what they may experience. Another way of engaging them with theory as the group progresses may be teaching notes after each group. Students could also be encouraged to reflect on their experience (Bandura, 1977) and on their group's process, perhaps writing this down in a personal diary.

At the outset, students were assigned to group rooms and each facilitator was allocated a list of students. Rooms and allotted times were adhered to throughout, although there were times when rooms were not vacated promptly or students were held up by previous classes. Sometimes furniture had to be moved, so the room could be transformed into the 'circle of chairs', the usual setting of the small group. The facilitators occasionally had to make sure that rooms were vacated on time by previous occupants.

All facilitators interpreted this activity to the groups as a metaphor to highlight their help to the students in carving out a space and a time for them in the institution.

Dynamic administration – is the group mandatory?

In a therapy situation, a group analytic psychotherapist would know her patients, their personal details and their circumstances. She would have control over her setting, the boundaries of the group, the time, the place and who would be coming. Ordinarily, she would interview each group member prior to inviting them into her therapeutic group, taking a diagnostic framework into consideration and drawing conclusions about how each new member might behave in the group. This aspect of the therapist's work is known as dynamic administration (Foulkes, 1964). A teacher would usually have a register to confirm attendance, even if she had not yet met all her students. The group facilitators, however, were somewhat at a loss, since at the beginning of the MSc course it had not yet been established whether group attendance was mandatory nor whether to record attendance.

Reflections and suggestions for future planning

Making the group mandatory is helpful in signalling its importance. Once a student has become a group member, that is after attendance in the first session, students who miss a group due to sickness or other reason will be 'missed' by their peers. Their absence changes the dynamics of the group and this is fed back to them upon their return. Leaving an empty chair for a missing member accentuates their absence and stresses the value of the members to each other. In large universities, it can be easy for students to feel unimportant and unseen. Valuing each single group members can be a particularly powerful experience for those who struggle with feelings of inadequacy and are unsure about their own worth.

The purpose of the group

Students are often unclear about the purpose of the experiential group. In any new teaching experience, including problem-based learning, the format and the purpose of coming together can seem obscure. Students often wait for directions and look to the facilitator for guidance.

Reflections and suggestions for future planning

In any new group rarely does anybody admit to knowing the purpose of the group. This is known as 'existential anxiety' and is a universal experience for any newcomer to any group (Yalom, 1985). This needs to be experienced to be appreciated and it often manifest in the silence that ensues once the group begins, particularly if the facilitator does not conform to usual classroom expectations and remains silent too.

In some of this MSc's experiential groups, students still do not know each other's names, even after one previous term together in seminars.

Reflections and suggestions

In some groups, a 'leader' may make themselves known by suggesting they introduce themselves (Bion, 1961). This often results in a reduction in anxiety, as does a declaration that someone feels anxious or uncomfortable. Self-reflection is the task in an experiential group (Bandura, 1977). Students tend to take on different roles in their groups quickly (Tubbs, 2011). Then the group as a whole can start to find its own way and explore the exciting possibilities a group can offer.

After the first experiential group, often two or three students drop out. It is difficult to encourage them back again, because often none of these students are as yet well known to the facilitator or their colleagues. Clearly the prospect of arriving in a group, a group with no apparent structure, was too daunting and confirms the necessity to provide some initial preparation for the students.

While the facilitator was told the number of students allocated, the first group attendances were patchy without a register. In good group analytic tradition, sufficient chairs were set up for all students and placed in a circle, and those students who attended observed the empty chairs of the students who were absent. Recognising this as a lack of coherence the attending students tried to encourage their fellow learners to be there the next time. Not having a register therefore gave the learners the power to decide as adults whether they attended or not, but also gave responsibility to a new community of practice (Wenger, 1998), here the group members in a precious, that is in terms of cost, experiential group.

We don't know what was said about the first group session outside the group, but the mystery of what went on during those ninety minutes seemed to have piqued the others' curiosity as attendance improved as time went on. The difficulty for the facilitators was the constrain of very few sessions, which meant that we had to work hard to engage the students quickly enough to allow them to gain from attending. The feedback from students was good, as the course directors increased the number of group sessions for the following year to ten.

Exploring students' difficulties

It was striking to hear about the difficulties some students had negotiating joining the course. Leaving behind families or children, making financial sacrifices and navigating a new city, and often all this in a second language. The university experience could easily have been similarly difficult had they not been given the opportunity to quickly bond with their peers. They gave and received support. When students arrive without a strong sense of belonging, this can be transformed quickly in the learning community. In a sensitively facilitated experiential group, these difficulties can be drawn out, addressed and ameliorated. Similarly a good, shared experience in a small group setting can bring students together emotionally, even more so when powerful emotional learning takes place. This can also occur when using simulation in a role play of potentially difficult situations, such as breaking bad news. If students learn to trust each other and see each other as a learning resource, they will be well-placed for future peer group learning and the kind of continuing professional development favoured by the GMC (General Medical Council).

Comparison with other models of small group teaching

In other kinds of small group teachings, like PBLs or clinical skills teaching (Gjibels et al., 2005) within the medical school, attendance is mandatory and a register is taken. The need for up to ninety percent attendance rate is ubiquitous in tertiary education but puts higher education teachers and facilitators into the often undesirable role of being authoritarian rather than assisting learners with their explorations (Jones, 2005). These two other settings are more structured than an experiential group, with clearly defined intended learning outcomes and the teacher acting as a kind of master of ceremonies. She ensures the material is covered, while students work through their tasks either using a handbook in the PBL, or instructions on how to examine the patient in a role play. She actively engages the students to introduce themselves to each other and uses their names. She establishes her credentials as expert in the field and in this way tacitly offers the understanding that she knows where the students need to go with their learning. She will be there to watch them execute it correctly – in her role of the 'midwife' (Jones, 2005). By asking Socratic questions, she gets them to engage with ideas and encourages them to contribute their own. 'Buzz' groups (Light and Cox, 2009) help, if the small group is dominated by shy people who have difficulty talking, or if the material is rather personal or anxiety provoking – for instance, when asking students to comment on matters of health, race, religion, gender or sexual orientation. Her friendly, non-judgemental style helps students to feel safe, to voice an opinion, try a role play or ask a question.

Students are generally eager to learn in an atmosphere that is encouraging and kind, when they get it wrong, but still usefully critical. They are helped to critique themselves and each other. Assessment and feedback is immediate. Skills are acquired and built on in the group (Bandura, 1977). The group task (Bion, 1961) is here explicitly to learn skills, but implicitly there is also learning to trust, gaining peer support and reflecting on one's own feelings about the material.

The experiential group is rather different as the facilitator says little. If asked questions directly about herself, she might respond that the group is anxious about her qualification for the role. This may evoke fleeting paranoid fears in the students that they are being set up or that they are in an experiment. They need to be allowed to reflect on these thoughts, on just how quickly anyone can become unsettled in unfamiliar territory. These are graduate students, not patients and yet they experience human vulnerability too.

When silent, the facilitator quickly becomes a receptacle for the students' projections. She will respond in a neutral but pleasant way – not unfriendly. Students who have experienced difficulties with authoritarian teachers may fear being judged or worry that the facilitator will feed back negative reports to the course directors. If they disclose personal material, they may worry about confidentiality and may start to organise the boundaries for themselves – defining rules for the group.

Reflections and suggestions for future planning

The facilitator will observe the behaviours and recall the communication both verbal and non-verbal and so models active listening. She may comment on it, describing the evidence of current anxieties reflected in these communications. In this way, the students get an opportunity to witness the work with unconscious processes being made conscious but will also experience being listened to in a deep way. Feeling heard is powerfully positive and helps reinforce the importance of using empathic understanding in working with patients.

When to present the theory

It is a valid question, if the lecture on groups and group therapy should be delivered before the experiential groups start. If students are presented with the theory of 'stages of the developmental life of a group' (Nitsun, 1989), they may miss the anxiety – for any newcomer – associated with the first session. The existential angst of wondering what they are supposed to do will be diluted, if this is described prior to the experience, since students will look out for it. Will this prevent them from the authentic first feelings that so powerfully link the new group experience to the experience of the 'microcosm of the social world'? (Foulkes, 1964). It usually fills us with dread and excitement simultaneously. If the facilitator acts similar to an ordinary teacher, will students develop the same intensity of attachment to them as to the 'person who has the answers'? The facilitator's role is two-fold, to help with reading the signs that appear in each of the students and make the learning explicit, but also as a container of that first anxiety.

Signposting unconscious material

If students focus on the minutiae of the coursework, rather than on the group process in the discussion during each experiential group, the question arises what they might be avoiding. Of course, there will be anxieties about the course and students' ability to complete it, particularly at times of assessments. But excessive preoccupation with it can be repetitive, ruminative and possibly an avoidance of other emotions. The facilitator might use Socratic questioning (Paul and Elder, 2006) to stimulate thoughts about the mental mechanisms that the students are taking refuge in and why. An apparently neutral discussion of examination questions may be a displacement activity of minds threatened with difficult or uncomfortable emotions, like fear of failure, envy of the clever student, shame at poor grades, pride in good grades, feeling ostracised by the group, feeling sexually attracted to forbidden others and so on.

The facilitator is a figure needed for safety, but she also controls the environment and therefore may be resented or rebelled against. She needs to be challenged, but not yet at the outset when everyone is still feeling too vulnerable. The group must find its own way first and the students eventually their own power. When they do, they will become less dependent on the facilitator, and more aware of the potential for creativity amongst the existing group members. This process of maturation and growing up is the most powerful experience of a well-functioning experiential group, earned through the exploration of individual identity and one's own potential as architect and navigator of one's own life and learning.

The ending

It is especially important to manage the ending of the group well. As previously mentioned, the students often come from far away and may have left parents or children behind in order to pursue their career. They have spent some profoundly intense times with their colleagues, who they have come to know in the group in a very different way from other university students and to whom they may have formed deep attachments.

Loss and separation are often experienced in a parallel process in the experiential group. Finishing a course and leaving an institution is a rite of passage that needs acknowledgement. It is a part of the teaching process to pick up these themes within the material of students' utterances – demonstrating to them the existence of unconscious mental mechanisms and linking their communications to their deeper feelings. This helps them to develop a greater awareness of themselves, their motives and their feelings. Self-reflection is positively reinforced (Schon, 1987) and so are any positive actions and attitudes that students demonstrate, in regard to themselves and towards each other. This is the altruism described by Yalom (1985), to be kind and considerate in this difficult task of continuous learning as adults throughout life.

Summary

Teaching and learning in small experiential groups provides the potential for deeper learning, as material can be presented in ways that encourages more active participation from the learner. The more emotional the impact on the students' experience, the more that experience will stay with them, if it is of a positive quality. In contrast, negative emotions can have a counterproductive effect on learning altogether. Inducing too much fear or anxiety may be discouraging, like the humiliating way of teaching in bygone days, or make the learners avoid attending altogether.

Of the three methods of small group teaching, PBLs are the most traditional and structured. They are useful in encouraging self-directed learning that can be directly observed and assessed by the teacher. The students learn to cooperate with each other and get a chance to try out different roles, particularly leading and chairing. They may be encouraged to facilitate other more quiet or non-contributing students. Clinical material impacts better with this style (Gjibels et al., 2005); however, this learning is less experiential, less emotive and possibly results in less retention of facts. The emotional sphere here might be enhanced by asking each member to use one word to describe their feelings about the clinical scenario in the PBL. Attaching emotion to a single word is quick and effective, as it induces impact on the limbic system, a part of the brain associated with deep learning.

Conclusion

The clinical skills teaching which is conducted in small groups lends itself well to simulation-based training. Small groups are emotionally a relatively safe environment, as ground rules are agreed and easy to secure. The use of role play with good actors enhances the learning experience and engages students in interesting scenarios. This presents a good balance of structured and experiential learning and is enjoyable as well as effective.

The small experiential group offers more experience than structure, but there are strategies that the facilitator can use to reduce adverse anxiety without diluting the experience. She can model empathic listening and deep observation. She can offer summaries at the end of each group and ask for feedback at the beginning of each next session.

In an experiential group, students need to be engaged early and quickly. This requires more active facilitation from the group leader than would normally be expected in a therapeutic group, but it reduces anxiety and makes it easier for vulnerable students to stay. Teaching of relevant theory before the group starts might be helpful and encourages engagement. Some carefully selected theoretical material could also be provided for the students outside of the group. Students can also be encouraged to keep a reflective log of their group experiences. Making attendance mandatory with an administrator taking a register and a strong commendation from the course directors to attend the experiential group may also ensure attendance. It may induce wavering students to turn up. Equally, support from the teaching faculty by ensuring prior seminars end on time and rooms are vacated promptly, sends signals of the value of the experiential group to the students and signifies that all staff are signed up to the process.

The tension between experience based and didactic teaching is an important one and deserves consideration. If the difference in value, quality and purpose is not addressed adequately and explained in detail, students may not be motivated to attend. They cannot learn from it, may not be able to value the experience and will not be competent or capable to use the relevant technique or method. All small group learning environments should be supported by teachers, who are emotionally literate and who can make the medium safe.

Chapter 18

Belonging

Inclusion and exclusion

Sue Einhorn

Introduction: when does a group become a gang?

I want to talk about belonging – about inclusion and exclusion, the power to include and exclude and the level of hidden violence attached to this theme within our society. The issues of inclusion and exclusion are the bread and butter of our work as group analysts and are offered as a challenge by Foulkes in his 'Basic Law of Group Dynamics', when he writes

> Group Members Collectively Constitute the very norm from which they Individually Deviate.
>
> (Foulkes, 1948, p. 29)

This is an ethical statement, as Dennis Brown said in his Foulkes Lecture (Brown, 1998), as well as an acknowledgement of the importance of groups in forming who we are.

I take it for granted that our individual self is constructed through the myriad of groups to which we belong. Belonging means groups that I 'take in' and which become part of my sense of self and give my life meaning. This is a continuing dynamic so that others who belong in the same group as me are also being constructed within that relationship. It is an ongoing interaction between us and all the members of the groups in which we participate. However, the co-construction of our self in a group setting and subject to the Basic Law of Group Dynamics suggests that the group norms facilitate each member to grow, and to be a separate and acceptable person, while also being a member, who enriches the culture of the group by contributing to the 'norms' of the group. What if the norms are those, for instance, of the current Hungary with barbed wire fences to keep refugees out? What if those who have power do not have the same ethical code as us?

Belonging

This lecture is about the complexity of belonging, especially as it is linked to exclusion and inclusion. However, the groups to which we belong mould

DOI: 10.4324/9781003310358-24

who we are, as we help to mould others, and however difficult they may be, give our lives colour and meaning. Let me begin then with a personal anecdote about the painful discussion of rejection/exclusion and our deeply felt need to feel included.

Many years ago, I went to university in a city a long way from London and found myself in a part of the UK that was beautiful and rural, but hostile to me. I was of the wrong class – the UK class system is embedded in a Royal Family, that is needed by the British hierarchy, and will survive whatever – had the wrong political attitudes, and needed to be taught what a girl should drink and how to behave in the pubs that my fellow students frequented, who were mostly landed upper class. In those days, I was a victim of their group, because I was threatened with exclusion if I did not fit in. To be accepted I had not only to learn their ways but also to agree that my differences could colour their lives but not seriously question or challenge them. To be accepted I had to submit and my discomfort with this unknown land – being a stranger there – meant that I became confused and hidden.

Why then was it so important to me, as a young woman, to be accepted? Why was it more important than being myself, so that myself began to be unacceptable to me? I felt ashamed and lonely. Being included at that time meant suppressing and rejecting a part of myself, but then it seemed more important to be accepted and included than to be myself. I am telling you this because inclusion can be as difficult as exclusion. Inclusion can be permeated with exclusion. What do I exclude of myself in order to be included, and what would have really happened had I not excluded those parts of myself? I wonder if this is linked to gender issues.

As we are relationship-seeking from our earliest days, we are groomed to this dialogue. The dialogue of learning that to be included we must identify with those, who have the power and to whom we must submit.

In a more open family a child will be able to influence the family, but primarily the family's values and customs will be inculcated into the child. David Glyn (Gyn, 2016, personal communication) described how we come to value ourselves. He gave a lovely, but painful example of a child having to adapt to family meals. These meals teach a child the social context of their family customs and this inevitably entails control over the child's own impulses. Family meals, he said, are a crucial area of the child's socialisation and lived introduction to the family's ideological values. Within the setting of the meal, the focus in terms of the interactions between child and others may fall on different issues, like how much the child eats, what the child eats, how the child behaves. Sitting still, wielding eating tools, verbal play or 'adult conversation'; or how a child manages the time frame of the meal, when eating with the family. There are few children for whom learning to participate in a meal does not entail considerable, apparently painful controls of bodily impulses, like for example suppressing the impulse to graze, using one's hands to eat or fingers to play with the interesting textures of the food. In negotiating or failing to negotiate this, the power dynamics of the family group are revealed. Who does and responds to what? What rules apply to whom? Where do the rules come from? The degree of rigidity with which the family group maintains its system of values will have an impact on the child's sense of its own value. But a child's sense of her own value also includes her ability to play a part in creating new values. In other words, is space being made for her? Does she feel welcomed into the family, or is she in the way?

It seems that in my university example, I valued being acceptable over valuing myself. This meant that I felt I had nothing to offer to this university group. My job was to become like them and exclude what I thought was unacceptable to them, because I was not sure if there was space for me.

The group life of the gang

Why is this dynamic so crucial and, as I would suggest, also part of everyone's experience? For example, as group analysts in the UK, we are included by some psychoanalytic groups but excluded by others. Are we analytic enough or are we too socially minded? As group analysts, we may exclude humanistically trained psychotherapists and see ourselves as superior to counsellors and may even demand that they see us as superior. The British class system is repeated throughout our psychoanalytic organisations.

As many have written, we are born relationship-seeking. To be part of and included in our family we have to learn the family group language, not just words but customs and hierarchy. From the earliest days a child has to learn to submit to the family or be regarded as 'the difficult one'. In fact, families often deal with the differences between family members by entitling them, 'the sensible one', 'the impossible one', 'the bossy one' and 'the sweet one'. You could say that to some extent small children are the victims of their families, because they have to curb their self-centredness in the interests of being acceptable to the family. We are groomed. We need to feel accepted, because if not, we feel isolated, frightened and very often shamed. To be unacceptable is to be shamed. Thus my submission to my university group shamed me, but my shame was expressed in mental confusion and body dysmorphia. This has to do with 'self-esteem'. If I am not acceptable as myself, then I must keep myself hidden, as the growing child has to keep herself hidden.

Scapegoating and gangs

The risk attached to not being included is not just to feel isolated and rejected but also carries the risk of being scapegoated. For some groups, particularly where there is violence, a group becomes a gang and is held together by focusing on who is unacceptable. Weakness and fear can be projected into a group member, who is then scapegoated and expelled. Here the extremes of belonging and rejection are most visible.

As group analysts, we understand that the person being scapegoated or expelled is part of a group dynamic and in this spirit, I would like to tell you about the coffee-bar I ran for street gangs in a New Town, and how the gangs dealt with inclusion and exclusion. What they taught me has been crucial to my work as a group analyst.

This was a youth project to provide a safe place for young people to meet. Gangs only make sense if members want to join or fear not belonging, since they live inclusion and exclusion as food for their very survival. The young people were aged between fourteen and twenty, and gang members rode motorbikes as noisily as possible to herald their arrival or departure. This noise was crucial to the sense of violence that permeated their lives.

In the 1960s and 1970s, there was a lot of writing about gangs in the UK as well as in the USA. These gangs were called 'unattached' youth, a famous example would be West Side Story. As youth workers, we were taught that the way to deal with these often quite anti-social groups of young people was to befriend the leader. The gang was beholden to the leader, who was either seen as the cleverest and most mature member or the most disturbed and violent member. He was bestowed with the power to protect or punish. The main purpose for these gangs was to protect their territory, sometimes to expand it, to defeat other gangs and to have a known headquarters that was their 'home from home'. Interestingly though, my coffee-bar became such a place for those too frightened to belong to a gang, although it was also protected by one of the gangs.

This was a town without work. Fathers were unemployed or absent, and mothers worked in the local biscuit factory. Violence was part of manhood, and each Saturday night, there would be fights in the town centre, often involving fathers and sons. Once a son could defeat his father, he came of age. A very macho environment that also affected the girls, but that is a separate story.

As we know, adolescence is a return to many of the emotional and psychological conflicts of childhood. Once again, a young person has to think about their own value. Having been valued at home does give a good start to being valued at school or by the peer group. However, adolescence is also such a powerful time, because the young person is also searching for a meaning to their life, for a purpose and, essentially, a place where they can make a contribution. For the street gangs, and for many of the other young people in this New Town, their fathers had lost their sense of purpose. There was a lot of drinking and fighting. In addition, the loss of jobs also heralded a changing world, where mining was redundant and new skills were needed. This community was on the 'slag heap' of a past society. Street corner fighting between gangs replaced the alienation and anomie of such an uncertain future. Prestige, status, meaning and excitement were located in the life of the gangs, because the wider world had left them confused and overwhelmed, unprepared for growing up. They were the scapegoats of a changing world and enacted their shame and humiliation, their anger and confusion, with and on each other. I should add that many of the more enterprising and confident young people sought economic advantage elsewhere. They went to more prosperous towns or emigrated to Australia or USA. The economic migrants we tend to exclude are often among some of the most enterprising.

Currently in the UK, the shamed and angry groups are the ones who have problems with immigrants, who they accuse of taking their jobs. The UK Brexit debate was riven with this. Did the UK survival depend on keeping 'them' out or us excluding ourselves from 'them'? Jo Joyce wrote to me that at one level, these groups think they are acting to 'protect' themselves, but as UK nationals they have more power than the immigrants they are targeting (Joyce, 2017, personal communication). Interestingly, some of the most vociferous voices wanting to keep immigrants out were recent immigrants themselves, but with UK status. There is a general sense of feeling threatened during 'austerity' and a fear that there is not enough to go around. As Foulkes says, our groups and ourselves are permeated to the core by the social context (Foulkes, 1964, p. 109). In other words, in this area where young men were excluded from employment and often from education as well, they enact their own exclusion by practising an extreme form of inclusion and exclusion through their gang life.

Anxiety

To elaborate all this need for leaders and scapegoats, I want to turn to Ernest Becker's book *The Denial of Death* (Becker, 2011). It acts as a foundation to much of what I am saying, but I am re-organising his arguments here. He basically says that as a species with self-consciousness and awareness, we are riven with anxiety, since the world is a terrifying place. This is increasingly more obvious as information pours in from every quarter of the world, ranging from natural disasters to man-made holocausts, but the most anxiety-provoking awareness is of our own mortality. As we awake to our living selves, we have to suppress the terrifying and inevitable knowledge of our own death. To quote Becker:

> This is the terror: to have emerged from nothing, to have a name, a consciousness of self, deep inner feelings, an excruciating inner yearning for life and self-expression – and with all this yet to die.
>
> (Becker, 2011, p. xii)

In our very earliest baby days, we are preoccupied with survival. When we are involved with the birth of a baby, we enter a unique time zone, where the miracle of this new baby becomes a highly sensitised moment. The utter dependence of the baby on its mother's body arouses extreme emotions of protectiveness and fear as well as a visceral love if all goes well. At a birth we are so close to its opposite, the risk of death. Will the baby survive? The responsibility for this new life brings overwhelming feelings to the new parents. The baby's task is to live, but the baby's birth has also brought the spectre of death. For a moment this risk exposes the underlying absurdity of life – we are born to die!

Not only do we have little control over society but we also certainly cannot control the fact that we are going to die. Of course, there are social differences. Women tend to live longer than men and, statistically, a more middle-class life often means a longer life, but all of us will die. How we deal with this fundamental anxiety is the subject of Becker's book, but also crucial for my argument it is what underlies our basic need to belong. We repress the anxiety about our mortality, it becomes our unconscious and we seek to find safety instead. For the street gangs this meant identifying with power. The gang and its leader became an exclusive, often closed group, although with rituals for joining, as for the fathers and their sons. Their search for meaning became preoccupied with defeating an enemy or needing to create an enemy and then defeating them, to avoid feeling the anxiety that an awareness of our own mortality can evoke. In other words, a tangible enemy such as a rival gang can be squashed, whereas death is intangible, and none of us know when or how it will catch up with us.

When you feel that you have little control over the little you have, focusing on a group that wants your territory or something else you have can be a relief. That other group has even less, it is lower in the power hierarchy, and can be demonised. The group norm in this situation does not allow for difference or individuality but demands a collective agreement that all differences need to be excluded. Differences arouse hostility and are projected outside the gang, onto the other gang or onto immigrants. Gangs have been known to unite in the excitement of identifying a common enemy!

Linking this with the massive refugee and asylum-seeking movement of people across Europe, we can see that people, who face death, are determined at any cost to find a new life. In the UK, rejecting an outsider group seems to make you feel more powerful than being able to influence the establishment. At the time, economic forces had put 'my' gangs at the bottom of the pecking order. It was easier for them to 'scapegoat' migrants, who themselves are victims of the economic order, while in fact both were 'victims' of powers beyond their control.

However, it is important here to include envy, an extremely destructive aspect of feeling excluded. Migrants and refugees have a second chance to build new lives. They come into a society new to them and have the chance to rebuild their lives if they can see the new society as a challenge with new opportunities for themselves and their children. This applied to the gangs too, since as I said before, many of the more confident young people attending my coffee-bar emigrated to other countries or to more prosperous parts of the UK. The oppressed locals in contrast felt unable to withstand the social changes they were living through. They saw themselves as deprived but also entitled to what they perceived others to have, which at the same time seemed beyond their reach, both economically and educationally. They simply did not have the confidence to go out into an often hostile world. Instead, they scapegoated the 'outsider' in the attempt to keep their own status, but also in order to deal with their envy of the migrant's mobility.

Conclusion

How does this link to our therapy groups? Groups not only construct who we become, and who we are always becoming, but they are also where we seek to either learn how to deal with the anxieties of living and/or protect ourselves from them. We need others to help build a sense of our own value but also to give our lives meaning and purpose. In agreement with Becker, groups are also an expression for the wish for the safety we felt as children, when family and community seemed eternal.

A group becomes a gang, when external anxieties dominate, and the group feels the need for a leader to rescue and to save them. Then the gang will find another group, onto which it can project all that is feared and try to defeat their fear by defeating that group.

Is this a long way from our therapy groups?

All group members experience the pain of feeling excluded in many of the sessions in which they participate. They have minority feelings. All group members seek to exclude certain behaviours or ideas to sustain their group culture. Feeling threatened and challenged activates these feelings, but they are of course essential, if people are to grow and change through group therapy. Members often join a group to change and then resist what that change entails, a basic fear of including difference (for example, homophobia).

In a mature group, there will be curiosity and interest in what new members bring, but also some fear and hostility about what will be demanded of them in opening up to a new group member. In a less mature or regressed group, there will be hostility, suspicion and a desire to exclude. Here will materialise all the issues mentioned above: rejection, aggression and the devaluing of what others bring.

The transference to the group conductor is important. Freud claimed that siblings actually hate each other but learn to love their siblings to keep their parents' love. A dilemma, when needing to manage envy, as well as wanting a more democratic ethos in the group. Gender differences are crucial.

In my experience, when the external world is in a particularly difficult state, belonging to a therapy group can be very harmonious because the hostility is out in the world.

Conclusion

Bibliography

Adorno, T. & Frankel-Brunswick, E. (2019) *The Authoritarian Personality*. London: Verso.

Akomfrah, J. (Director) (2012) *The Unfinished Conversations* [Film]. UK: Tate. Available at: https://www.youtube.com/watch?v=F4-ktD5I_Sc

Anthony, J. (1988) 'The Dilemma of Therapeutic Leadership: The Leader Who Does Not Lead'. In Tuttman, S. (ed.) *Psychoanalytic Group Theory and Therapy: Essays in Honour of Saul Scheidlinger*. Madison, CT: International University Press, pp. 71–86.

Appignanesi, L. (2008) *Mad, Bad and Sad: A History of Women and the Mind Doctors from 1800 to the Present*. London: Virago Press.

Azu-Okeke, O. (1993) 'Conflict in the Search for an 'Individual Self' as Opposed to a Traditional 'Group Self': A Consequence of Undertaking Group-Analytic Training'. *Group Analysis* 26(3): 261–268.

Bagilishya, D. (2000) 'Mourning and Recovering from Trauma in Rwanda, Tears Flowin'. *Transcultural Psychiatry*, September 2000. Available at: https://changingthestory.leeds.ac.uk/2020/03/19/making-connections-reflections-on-the-use-of-proverbs-in-research-and-practice/

Bandura, A. (1977) *Social Learning Theory*. New York: General Learning Press.

Barnes, E. (ed.) (1968) *Psychosocial Nursing*. London: Tavistock.

Barnett, B. (2007) *"You Ought To!" A Psychoanalytic Study of the Superego and Conscience*. London: Karnac.

Barwick, N. & Weegman, M. (2017) *Group Therapy – A Group-Analytic Approach*. London: Routledge.

Bateman, A. & Fonagey, P. (2006) *Mentalization-Based Treatment for Borderline Personality Disorder*. Oxford: Oxford University Press.

Beck, W. (2015) 'Group Analysis in China—Challenges in a Changing Society'. *Group Analysis* 48(2): 164–173.

Becker, E. (2011) *The Denial of Death*. New York: Souvenir Press.

Beckett, S. (1958) *Endgame*. New York: Grove Press.

Behr, H. & Hearst, L. (2005) *Group Analytic Psychotherapy*. London: Whurr.

Benjamin, J. (2018) *Beyond Doer and Done To: Recognition Theory, Intersubjectivity and the Third*. London: Routledge.

Berman, A. & Weinberg, H. (1998) 'The Advanced Stage Therapy Group'. *International Journal of Group Psychotherapy* 48(4): 499–518.

Biggs, J. B. (1987) *Student Approaches to Learning and Studying*. Hawthorn, VIC: Australian Council for Educational Research.

Bion, W. R. (1961) *Experiences in Groups*. London: Tavistock.

Bion, W. R. (1962) *Learning from Experience*. London: Heinemann.

Blackwell, D. (1997) 'Holding, Containing and Bearing Witness: The Problem of Helpfulness in Encounters with Torture Survivors'. *Journal of Social Work Practice* 11(2): 81–89.

Blackwell, D. (2002) 'Out of Their Class: Class, Colonization and Resistance in Analytic Psychotherapy and Group Analysis'. *Group Analysis* 35(3): 367–380.

Bledin, K. (2003) 'Migration, Identity and Group Analysis'. *Group Analysis* 36(1): 97–110.

Bollas, C. (1990) 'The Fascist State of Mind'. In *Being a Character*. London: Routledge, pp. 193–217.

Boyd, J. (1991) 'Facilitating Personal Transformations in Small Groups'. In Boyd, R. (ed.) *Personal Transformations in Groups: A Jungian Perspective*. London and New York: Routledge.

Britton, R. (1999) *Sex, Death and the Superego*. London: Karnac.

Brown, D. & Pedder, J. (1987) *Introduction to Psychotherapy: An Outline of Psychodynamic Principles and Practice*. London: Routledge.

Brown, D. (1992a) 'Transcultural Group Analysis I. Different Views of Maastricht and Heidelberg'. *Group Analysis* 25(1): 87–96.

Brown, D. (1992b) 'Transcultural Group Analysis II. Use and Abuse of Cultural Differences: Analysis and Ethics'. *Group Analysis* 25(1): 97–105.

Brown, D. & Zinkin, L. (1993) *The Psyche and the Social World: Developments in Group-Analytic Theory*. The International Library of Group Psychotherapy and Group Process. London and New York: Routledge.

Brown, D. (1998) 'Foulkes Lecture 1998'. *Group Analysis* 31: 391–420.

Brown, D. (2001) 'A Contribution to the Understanding of the Social Unconscious'. *Group Analysis* 34(1): 29–38.

Brown, D. (2006) *Resonance and Reciprocity*. London: Routledge.

Buddhist Sutras, Lulu (tarns), 1987.

Burkitt, I. (1991) 'Power Relations, Interdependencies and Civilized Personality'. In Phillips, K. (ed.) *Social Selves*. London: Sage, pp. 163–188.

Burman, E. (2002) 'Gender, Sexuality and Power in Groups'. *Group Analysis* 35(4): 540–559.

Burns, A. (2018) *Milkman*. London: Faber & Faber.

Butler, J. (2004) *Precarious Life: The Power of Mourning and Violence*. New York and London: Verso Books.

Chen, E. C., Kakkad, D. & Balzano, J. (2008) 'Multicultural Competence and Evidence-Based Practice in Group Therapy'. *Journal of Clinical Psychology* 64(11): 1261–1278.

Claremont de Castillejo, I. (1974) *Knowing Woman*. New York and London: Harper Colophon.

Clark, M. A., Anand, V. & Roberson, L. (2000) 'Resolving Meaning: Interpretation in Diverse Decision-Making Groups'. *Group Dynamics: Theory, Research, and Practice* 4: 211–221.

Collins Dictionary (1999) London and Glasgow: Collins.

Crépeau, P. & Bizimana, S. (1979) *Proverbes du Rwanda*. Tervuren: Musée Royal de l'Afrique Centrale.

Dalal, F. (1998) *Taking the Group Seriously: Towards a Post-Foulkesian Group Analytic Theory.* London: Jessica Kingsley.

Dalal, F. (2001) 'The Social Unconscious: A Post-Foulkesian Perspective'. *Group Analysis* 34(4): 539–555.

Dalal, F. (2002) *Race, Colour and the Processes of Racialisation.* London: Routledge.

David, M. (2016) 'The Group Analyst's Role When Facing the Group'. *Group Analysis* May 23.

Davis, H. (2004) *Understanding Stuart Hall.* London: Sage.

Devan, G. S. (2001) 'Culture and the Practice of Group Psychotherapy in Singapore'. *International Journal of Group Psychotherapy* 51(4): 571.

Dizadji, F. (2016) *Trauma and Refugees* (unpublished).

Edmundson, M. (2007) *The Death of Sigmund Freud – Facism, Psychoanalysis and the Rise of Fundamentalism.* London: Bloomsbury.

Einhorn, S. (2007) Transmission of Trauma: Response to Lecture by Gerhard Wilke'. *Group Analysis*, 40(4): 457–463.

Einhorn, S. (2018) *Countertransference in Groups* (unpublished).

Elias, N. (1978) *What Is Sociology?* New York: Columbia University Press.

Elias, N. (1994) (trans E. Jephcott) *The Civilising Process.* Oxford: Blackwells.

Erikson, E. (1966) 'Eight Ages of Man'. *International Journal Psycho-Analysis* 47: 281–300.

Evans, S. (1998) 'Beyond the Mirror: A Group-Analytic Exploration of Late Life and Depression'. *Aging & Mental Health* 2(2): 94–99.

Ezriel, H. (1972) 'Experimentation within the Psychoanalytic Session'. *Contemporary Psychoanalysis* 8: 229–245.

Ezriel, H. (1980) 'A Psychoanalytic Approach to Group Treatment'. In Scheidlinger, pp. 109–146.

Figueira, S. A. (1991) 'On Being a Psychoanalyst in Brazil: Pressures, Pitfalls and Perspectives'. *Free Associations* 2(3): 423–446.

Foucault, M. (1992) 'The Subject and Power'. In Ingram, D. & Simon-Ingram, J. (eds.) *Critical Theory: The Essential Readings.* St. Paul, MN: Paragon House.

Foulkes, E. (ed.) (1990) *Selected Papers of S.H.Foulkes: Psychoanalysis and Group Analysis.* London: Karnac.

Foulkes, S. H. (1948) *Introduction to Group-Analytic Psychotherapy.* London: Heinemann.

Foulkes, S. H. & Anthony, E. J. (1957) *Group Psychotherapy: The Psychoanalytic Approach.* London: Maresfield Reprints.

Foulkes, S. H. (1964) *Therapeutic Group Analysis.* London: George Allen and Unwin.

Foulkes, S. H. (1964a) 'Concerning Leadership'. *Therapeutic Group Analysis.* London: Allen & Unwin.

Foulkes, S. H. (1964b) 'Group Analysis in a Military Neurosis Centre'. In *Therapeutic Group Analysis.* London: George Allen & Unwin, pp. 187–193.

Foulkes, S. H. (1964c) 'A Brief Guide to Group-Analytic Theory and Practice'. In *Therapeutic Group Analysis.* London: George Allen & Unwin, pp. 281–310.

Foulkes, S. H. (1971) 'Access to Unconscious Processes in the Group-Analytic Group'. In Foulkes, E. (ed.) *Selected Papers: Psychoanalysis and Group Analysis.* London: Karnac Books (1990).

Foulkes, S. H. (1973) 'The Group as Matrix of the Individual's Mental Life'. In Wolberg, L. R. & Schwartz, E. K. (eds.) *Group Therapy.* New York: Intercontinental Medical Books.

Foulkes, S. H. (1975) 'The Leader in the Group'. In Foulkes, E. (ed.) *Selected Papers of S. H. Foulkes Psychoanalysis and Group Analysis*. London: Karnac.

Foulkes, S. H. & Anthony, E. (1984) *Group Psychotherapy: The Psychoanalytic Approach*. London: Karnac.

Foulkes, S. H. (1986) *Group Analytic Psychotherapy. Methods and Principles*. London: Karnac.

Foulkes, S. H. (1990) 'The Leader in the Group'. In *Selected Papers*. London: Karnac, pp. 285–296.

Foulkes, S. H. (1991) *Group-Analytic Psychotherapy, Methods and Principles*. London: Karnac Books.

Fraiberg, S., Adelson, E. & Shapiro, V. (1975) 'Ghosts in the Nursery'. *Journal of the American Academy of Child Psychiatry* 14(3): 387–421.

Frankfurt Institute for Social Research (1973) *Aspects of Sociology*. London: Heinemann.

Freud, S. (1915) *The Unconscious*. SE Vol XIV.

Freud, S. (1917) 'Mourning and Melancholia'. *Collected Papers*. London: Macmillan GPT.

Freud, S. (1921/1985) 'Group Psychology and the Analysis of the Ego'. In Richards, A. & Dickson, A. (eds.) *The Penguin Freud Library Vol 12*. Penguin: London.

Freud, S. (1926) 'Inhibitions, Symptoms and Anxiety'. *New Introductory Lectures* SE, 16.

Freud, S. (1996) *Moses and Monotheism*. New York: Random House.

Freud, S. & Freud, A. (2001) '"An Autobiographical Study", "Inhibitions", "Symptoms and Anxiety", "Lay Analysis" and Other Works'. *SE*, 20.

Fromm, E. (1970) *The Crisis of Psychoanalysis: Essays on Freud, Marx and Social Psychology*. London: Penguin.

Fromm, E. (1995) *The Art of Loving*. London: Thorsons.

Fromm, E. (1997) *The Anatomy of Human Destructiveness*. London: Pimlico.

Fromm, E. (1999) 'The Social Unconscious'. Ch. 10 in *The Erich Fromm Reader: Readings Selected and Edited by Rainer Funk*. New York: Humanity Books.

Frosh, S. (2009) 'Where Did Class Go? Psychoanalysis and Social Identities'. *Sitegeist* 3: 99–116.

Garland, C. (1982) 'Taking the Non-Problem Seriously'. *Group Analysis* 15(1): 4–14.

Gjibels, D., Docht, F., Van der Bosch, P. & Segers, M. (2005) 'Effects of a Problem-Based Learning: A Meta-Analysis from the Angle of Assessment'. *Review of Educational Research* 75(1): 27–61.

Gourevitch, P. (to be published 2023) *You Hide That You Hate Me, I Hide That I Know*. New York: Farrar, Straus and Giroux.

Gramsci, A. & Forgacs, D. (1999) *The Gramsci Reader: Selected Writings, 1916–1935*. London: Lawrence and Wishart.

Harrison, T. (2000) *Bion, Rickman, Foulkes and the Northfield Experiments: Advance on a Different Front*. London: Jessica Kingsley.

Hesse, B. (2000) *Un/settled Multiculturalisms*. London: Zed Books.

Heaney, S. (1975) *North*. London: Faber and Faber.

Hinshelwood, R. D. (2008) 'Group Therapy as Psychic Containing'. *International Journal of Group Psychotherapy* 58(3): 283–302.

Holy Bible (AV) (1662) Oxford: Oxford University Press.

Hopper, E. (1996) 'The Social Unconscious in Clinical Work'. *Group* 20(1): 7–42.

Hopper, E. (2000) 'From Objects and Subjects to Citizens: Group Analysis and the Study of Maturity'. *Group Analysis* 33: 29–34.

Hopper, E. (2003a) *The Social Unconscious: Selected Papers*. London: Karnac.

Hopper, E. (2003b) *Traumatic Experience in the Unconscious Life of Groups*. London: Jessica Kingsley.

Hopper, E. (ed) (2012) *Trauma and Organisations*. London: Karnac.

Horne, A. (1992) 'Control and Leadership in Group Psychotherapy'. *Group Analysis* 25: 2.

Hornstein, G. (2000) *To Redeem One Person is to Redeem the World: The Life of Frieda Fromm-Reichman*. New York: Free Press.

Hutchinson, S. (2009) 'Foulkesian Authority: Another View. Response to Lecture by Morris Nitsun'. *Group Analysis* 42: 354.

Jacoby, R. (1975) *Social Amnesia*. Sussex: Harvester Press.

James, C. (1982a) *Bion's "Containing" and Winnicott's "Holding" in the Context of the Group Matrix*. Published online 2015.

James, C. (1982b) 'Transitional Phenomena and the Matrix in Group Psychotherapy'. In Pines, M. et al. (eds.) *The Individual and the Group*. New York: Plenum Press.

James, J. & Joyce, A. (2015) *The Practice of Psychoanalytic Parent-Infant Psychotherapy: Claiming the Baby*. 2nd edn. London: Routledge.

James, J. (2016) 'Parent–Infant Psychotherapy in Groups'. In Baradon, T., Biseo, M., Broughton, C., James, J., & Joyce, A. (eds.) *The Practice of Psychoanalytic Parent–Infant Psychotherapy, Claiming the Baby*. London: Routledge.

Jones, A. (2006) 'Levels of Change in Parent-Infant Psychotherapy'. *Journal of Child Psychotherapy* 32(3): 295–311.

Jones, G. (2005) 'Gatekeepers, Midwives and Fellow Travellers'. In *Gatekeepers, Midwives and Fellow Travellers: The Craft and Artistry of Adult Educators*. London: Mary Ward Centre, pp. 5–16.

Joyce, J. (1922/1960) *Ulysses*. London: Bodley Head.

Jung, C. (1950) 'Concerning Mandala Symbolism'. In Read, H., Fordham, M., Adler, G., & McGuire, W. (eds.) *The Archetypes and the Collective Unconscious*. Collected Works, Vol. 9:1. London: Routledge and Kegan Paul, pp. 355–384.

Jung, C. G. (1955) 'The Conjunction'. In Fordham, M., Adler, G., & Mcguire, W. (eds.) *Mysterium Coniunctionis*. Collected Works, Vol. 14. London: Routledge and Kegan Paul, pp. 457–553.

Jung, C. G. (1974) *Psychology and Alchemy*. In Collected Works, Vol. 12. London: Routledge & Kegan Paul.

Jung, C. G. (1977) *The Relations between the Ego and the Unconscious*. Collected Works Vol. 7. London: Routledge & Kegan Paul.

Kinzie, J. D., Leung, P., Bui, A., Ben, R., Keopraseuth, K. O., Riley, C., Fleck, J. & Ades, M. (1988) 'Group Therapy with Southeast Asian Refugees'. *Community Mental Health Journal* 24(2): 157–166.

Kohut, H. & Wolf, E. S. (1978) 'The Disorders of the Self and their Treatment: An Outline'. *International Journal of Psychoanalysis* 59(4): 413–425.

Kolb, D. A. (1984) *Experiential Learning: Experience as the Source of Learning and Development*. Englewood Cliffs, NJ: Prentice Hall.

Kotani, H. (1999) 'Aspects of Intrapsychic, Interpersonal and Cross-Cultural Dynamics in Japanese Group Psychotherapy'. *International Journal of Group Psychotherapy* 49(1): 93–104.

Laplanche, J. (1999) 'The Unfinished Copernican Revolution'. In *Essays on Otherness*. London: Routledge (translated by J. Fletcher), pp. 53–85.

Le Roy, J. (1994) 'Group Analysis and Culture'. In Brown, D., & Zinkin, L. (eds.) *The Psyche and the Social World*. London: Routledge, pp. 180–201.

Lieberman, A. F., Padrón, E., Van Horn, P. & Harris, W. W. (2005) 'Angels in the Nursery: The Intergenerational Transmission of Benevolent Parental Influences'. *Infant Mental Health Journal* 26(6): 504–520.

Light, G. & Cox, R. (2009) 'Facilitating Small Group Teaching'. In *Learning and Teaching in Higher Education*. London: Sage, pp. 127–153.

Lorentzen, S., Maar, V. & Sørlie, T. (2006) 'A Training Program in Group Analysis in the Baltic States: Six Years' Experience'. *Group Analysis* 39(4): 494–516.

Loudis, J. (2017) 'Editor's Note'. *World Policy Journal* 34(4): 1–2.

MacGregor, C. (2012) 'Matrix and Patrix: The Conductor, The Group and The Parental Dyad. In Review of the International Summer Conference "Different Homes for Group Analysis" in Lithuania'. *Group-Analytic Contexts* December 2012 No. 58.

Malan, D. (1979) *Individual Psychotherapy and the Science of Psychodynamics*. London: Butterworths.

Manning, N. (1989) *The Therapeutic Community: Charisma and Routinisation*. London: Routledge.

Maquet, J. (1961) *The Premise of Inequality in Ruanda*. London: Oxford University Press.

Marcuse, H. (1962) *Eros and Civilisation*. New York: Vintage.

Marcuse, H. (2002) *One Dimensional Man*. London and New York: Routledge.

Martinon, J.-P. (2006) *Rwandan Proverbs*. Available at: https://jeanpaulmartinon.net/rap/rwanda/rwanda-proverbs/

Marx, K. (1974) *Das Kapital: A Critique of Political Economy*. London: Lawrence and Wishart.

Masson, J. (1985) *Complete Letters of Sigmund Freud to W. Fliess (1887–1904)*. Cambridge, MA: Harvard University Press.

McGilchrist, I. (2009) *The Master and His Emissary*. London: Yale University Press.

McNeill, D. G. Jr. (2002) 'Killer Songs'. *The New York Times* March 17, 2002.

Menzies Lyth, I. E. P. (1960) 'A Case-Study in the Functioning of Social Systems as a Defence against Anxiety'. *Human Relations* 13(2): 95–121.

Mitchell, J. (1974) *Psychoanalysis and Feminism*. London: Allen Lane.

Monbiot, G. (2018) *Out of the Wreckage: A New Politics for an Age of Crisis*. London and New York: Verso.

Nitsun, M. (1989) 'Early Development: Linking the Individual and the Group'. *Group Analysis* 22(3): 249–261.

Nitsun, M. (1996) *The Anti-Group: Destructive Forces in the Group and Their Therapeutic Potential*. London: Routledge.

Nitsun, M. (2009) 'Authority and Revolt: The Challenges of Group Leadership'. *Group Analysis* 42: 325.

Nitsun, M. (2014) *Beyond the Anti-Group: Survival and Transformation*. London: Routledge.

Nitzgen, D. (2001) 'Training in Democracy, Democracy in Training: Notes on Group Analysis and Democracy'. *Group Analysis* 34: 331.

Nitzgen, D. (2016) 'Reflections on Group Analysis and Philosophy'. *Group Analysis* 49: 1.

Noack, A. (2002a) 'Working with Trainees in Experiential Groups'. In Chesner, A. & Hahn, H. (eds.) *Creative Advances in Groupwork*. London: Jessica Kingsley.

Noack, A. (2002b) *Regression, Integration and the Acceptance of Limitations.* (unpublished).

Ogden, T. H. (1989) *The Primitive Edge of Experience*. London: Karnac.

Paul, R. & Elder, L. (2006) *The Art of Socratic Questioning*. Dillon Beach, CA: Foundation for Critical Thinking.

Pells, K., Breed, A., Uwihoreye, C. et al. (2021) 'No-One Can Tell a Story Better than the One Who Lived It': Reworking Constructions of Childhood and Trauma Through the Arts in Rwanda'. *Culture, Medicine and Psychiatry*. Available at: https://doi.org/10.1007/s11013-021-09760-3

Pines, M. (1982) *The Evolution of Group Analysis*. London: RKP.

Pines, M. (1985) *Bion and Group Psychotherapy*. London: RKP.

Pines, M. (1998) 'Group Analytic Psychotherapy and the Borderline Patient'. In *Circular Reflections*. London: Jessica Kingsley.

Powell, A. (1989) 'The Nature of the Group Matrix'. *Group Analysis* 22(3): 271–281.

Powell, A. (1990) 'Words and Music: An Unsung Therapeutic Alliance'. *Group Analysis* 23(3): 225–235.

Powell, A. (1991a) 'Matrix, Mind and Matter: From the Internal to the Eternal'. *Group Analysis* 24(3): 299–322.

Powell, A. (1991b) 'The Embodied Matrix: Discussion on Paper by Romano Fiumara'. *Group Analysis* 24(4): 419–423.

Powell, A. (1992) 'The Concept of Matrix – A Metaphysical Enquiry'. *Group Analysis* 25(1): 107–113.

Powell, A. (1993) 'The Psychophysical Matrix and Group Analysis'. *Group Analysis* 26(4): 449–468.

Prodgers, A. (1990) 'The Dual Nature of the Group as Mother: The Uroboric Container'. *Group Analysis* 23(1): 17–23.

Reck, A. J. (1964) *Selected Writings: George Herbert Mead*. Chicago, IL: Chicago University Press.

Rohlfing, S. et al. (2014) 'Das Geschlecht in der Gruppe oder Das Geschlecht der Gruppe? "Doing Gender" in der Gruppenpsychotherapie'. *Gruppenpsychotherapie + Gruppendynamik* 50(3): 190–218.

Rohr, E. (2002) 'Lost Shadows – Migrants, Refugees and Social Class: A Group-Analytic Challenge'. *Group Analysis* 35(3): 424–436.

Rohr, E. (2014) 'Intimacy and Social Suffering in a Globalised World'. *Group Analysis* 47(4): 365–383.

Rouchy, J. P. (1995) 'Identification and Groups of Belonging'. *Group Analysis* 28(2): 129–142.

Ruddock, J. (1978) 'Learning Through Small Group Discussion'. In *Research into Higher Education Monographs*. Guilford: University of Surrey.

Ryan, J. (2017) *Psychoanalysis and Class: The Psychic Landscapes of Inequality*. London: Routledge.

Scheidlinger, S. (ed.) (1980) *Psychoanalytic Group Dynamics*. New York: International Universities Press.

Schlapobersky, J. (2016) *From the Couch to the Circle*. London: Routledge.

Schon, D. A. (1987) *Educating the Reflective Practitioner; Toward a New Design for Teaching and Learning in the Professions*. San Francisco, CA: Jossey-Bass.

Searles, H. (1986a) *Collected Papers on Schizophrenia and Related Subjects.* London: Karnac.

Searles, H. (1986b) *Collected Papers.* London: Karnac.

Sengun, S. (1997) 'What Is Therapeutic and What Is Cultural? Discussion of Paper by Friedhelm Roder and Petar Opalic'. *Group Analysis* 30(2): 241–243.

Sengun, S. (2001) 'Migration as a Transitional Space and Group Analysis'. *Group Analysis* 34: 65–78.

Sengun, S. (2003) 'Discussion on 'The Culture of the Group and Groups from Different Cultures' by Haim Weinberg'. *Group Analysis* 36(2): 268–273.

Skynner, R. (1976) *One Flesh: Separate Persons.* London: Constable.

Slade, A. (2005) 'Parental Reflective Functioning: An Introduction'. *Attachment & Human Development* 7(3): 269–281.

Stacey, R. D. (2000) 'Reflexivity, Self Organisation and Emergence in the Group Matrix'. *Group Analysis* 33(4): 501.

Stacey, R. D. (2001) 'Complexity and the Group Matrix', cited in Dalal, F. (2001) 'The Social Unconscious'. *Group Analysis* 34(2): 221–239.

Steiner, J. (1993) *Psychic Retreats.* London: Routledge.

Steuer, J. L., Mintz, I., Hammen, C. L., Hill, M. A., Jarvik, L. F., McCraley, T., Motoike, P., Rosen, R. et al. (1984) 'Cognitive-Behavioural and Psychodynamic Group Therapy in the Treatment of Geriatric Depression'. *Journal of Consult & Clinic Psychology* 52(2): 180–109.

Storck, L. (2002) 'Editorial Introduction'. *Group Analysis: Special Edition: A Group Analysis of Class, Status Groups and Inequality* 35(3): 39–41.

Szasz, T. (1973) *Ideology and Insanity.* London: Penguin Press.

Taha, M., Mahfouz, R. & Arafa, M. (2008) 'Socio-Cultural Influence on Group Therapy Leadership Style'. *Group Analysis* December, 41(4): 391–406.

Thatcher, M. (1987) *Thatcher Archive* (THCR 5/2/.262): COI transcript. Also in *Women's Own* October 31, pp. 8–10.

Trist, E. & Murray H. (ed.) (1990) *The Social Engagement of Social Science, Vol. 1. The Social-Psychological Perspective.* London: Free Associations.

Tsui, P. & Schultz, G. L. (1988) 'Ethnic Factors in Group Process: Cultural Dynamics in Multi-Ethnic Therapy Groups'. *American Journal of Orthopsychiatry* 58(1): 136–142.

Tubbs, S. L. (2011) *A Systems Approach to Small Group Interaction.* 11th ed. New York: Random House.

Turkle, S. (2011) *Alone Together: Why We Expect More from Technology and Less from Each Other.* New York: Basic Books.

Turkle, S. TED talk 2013.

University of Manitoba, Canada, Anthropology course notes. (visited on 3.5.2019) Available at: https://www.umanitoba.ca/faculties/arts/anthropology/courses/122/module1/social.html

Uwihoreye, C. & Pells, K. (2020) *Leeds University – Changing the Story – Making Connections: Reflections on the Use of Proverbs in Research and Practice.* (visited on 19.03.2020) Available at: https://changingthestory.leeds.ac.uk/

Van der Kleij, G. (1985) 'The Group and Its Matrix'. *Group Analysis* 18(2): 102–110.

van Schoor, E. (1997) 'Socio-Cultural Aspects of British and American Group Psychotherapy'. *Group Analysis* 30(1): 27–43.

Vincent, D. (2016) 'Couple and Family Dynamics and Triangular Space in Group Psychotherapy'. In Novakovic, A. (ed.) *Couple Dynamics*. London: Karnac, pp. 124–125.

Weinberg, H. (2003) 'The Culture of the Group and Groups from Different Cultures'. *Group Analysis* 36(2): 253–268.

Wenger, E. (1998) *Communities of Practice; Learning, Meaning and Identity*. Cambridge: Cambridge University Press, pp. 3–11.

Whitford, M. (1991) *Luce Irigary, Philosophy in the Feminine*. London: Routledge.

Wilke, G. (2007) 'Foulkes Lecture 2007'. *Group Analysis* 38: 429–447.

Wilke, G. (2014) *The Art of Group Analysis in Organisations*. London: Karnac.

Winnicott, D. W. (1945) 'Primitive Emotional Development'. In Khan, M. (ed.) *Through Paediatrics to Psychoanalysis: Collected Papers* 1958. London: Tavistock, pp. 145–156.

Winnicott, D. W. (1953) *Playing and Reality*. London and New York: Routledge, 2012.

Winnicott, D. W. (1958) 'The Capacity to be Alone'. In Sutherland, J. D. (ed.) *The Maturational Process and the Facilitating Environment* (1965). London: Hogarth Press, pp. 29–36.

Winnicott, D. W. (1974) *Playing and Reality*. London: Penguin.

Wood, H. (2007) *Compulsive Use of Virtual Sex and Internet Pornography: Addiction or Perversion?* London: Karnac.

Yalom, I. D. (1985) *The Theory and Practice of Group Psychotherapy*. Chapter 1. New York: Therapeutic Factors in Groups.

Yamaguchi, T. (1986) 'Group Psychotherapy in Japan Today'. *International Journal of Group Psychotherapy* 36(4): 567–578.

Zinkin, L. (1989) 'A Gnostic View of the Therapy Group'. *Group Analysis* 22(2): 201–217.

Zinkin, L. (1998) *Dialogue in the Analytic Setting*. London: Jessica Kingsley.

Index